Short-Term Dynamic Psychotherapy

CLINICAL INSIGHTS

CLINICAL AND RESEARCH ISSUES IN

Short-Term Dynamic Psychotherapy

Edited by
ARNOLD WINSTON, M.D.

Director, Department of Psychiatry,
Beth Israel Medical Center; and
Professor of Clinical Psychiatry,
Mount Sinai School of Medicine,
City University of New York

AMERICAN PSYCHIATRIC PRESS, INC.
Washington, D.C.

Note: The authors have worked to ensure that all information in this book concerning drug dosages, schedules, and routes of administration is accurate at the time of publication and consistent with standards set by the U.S. Food and Drug Administration and the general medical community. As medical research and practice advance, however, therapeutic standards may change. For this reason and because human and mechanical errors sometimes occur, we recommend that readers follow the advice of a physician directly involved in their care or the care of a member of their family.

Library of Congress Cataloging in Publication Data

Main entry under title:

Clinical and research issues in short-term dynamic psychotherapy.

Based on a symposium on short-term dynamic psychotherapy presented at the American Psychiatric Association Meeting in May 1984.
Half-title: Short-term dynamic psychotherapy.
Includes bibliographies.
I. Psychotherapy, Brief—Congresses. I. Winston, Arnold, 1935-
II. American Psychiatric Association. Meeting (137th : 1984 : Los Angeles, Calif.) III. Title: Short-term dynamic psychotherapy. [DNLM:
1. Psychotherapy, Brief—Congresses.
WM 420 C6405 1984]
RC480.55.C48 1985 616.89'14 84-28276
ISBN 0-88048-072-6 (pbk.)

Printed in the U.S.A.

Contents

Contributors

Harold Been, M.D.
Physician-in-Charge, Center for Teaching and Research in Short-Term Dynamic Psychotherapy, Department of Psychiatry, Beth Israel Medical Center; and Senior Clinical Instructor, Mount Sinai School of Medicine, City University of New York

Victor Goldin, M.D.
Associate Director for Education, Department of Psychiatry, Beth Israel Medical Center; and Assistant Professor of Clinical Psychiatry, City University of New York

Althea Horner, Ph.D.
Consulting Psychologist, Department of Psychiatry, Beth Israel Medical Center

Leigh McCullough, Ph.D.
Research Associate, Department of Psychiatry, Beth Israel Medical Center; and Clinical Instructor, Mount Sinai School of Medicine, City University of New York

Peggy Nepps, Psy.D.
Supervising Psychologist, Department of Psychiatry, Beth Israel Medical Center; and Instructor, Mount Sinai School of Medicine, City University of New York

Henry Pinsker, M.D.
Associate Director, Department of Psychiatry, Beth Israel Medical Center; and Associate Professor of Clinical Psychiatry, Mount Sinai School of Medicine, City University of New York

Jerome Pollack, M.D.
Physician-in-Charge, Brief Adaptation-Oriented Psychotherapy, Department of Psychiatry, Beth Israel Medical Center; and Assistant Clinical Professor of Psychiatry, Mount Sinai School of Medicine, City University of New York

Joel Redfield, Ph.D.
Chief Psychologist, Department of Psychiatry, Beth Israel Medical Center; and Assistant Professor of Psychiatry, Mount Sinai School of Medicine, City University of New York

ISABEL SKLAR, M.S.W.
Associate Director, Department of Social Work, Beth Israel Medical Center; and Teaching Associate, Departments of Psychiatry and Community Medicine, Mount Sinai School of Medicine, City University of New York

MANUEL TRUJILLO, M.D.
Physician-in-Charge, Research and Program Evaluation, Department of Psychiatry, Beth Israel Medical Center; and Assistant Professor of Clinical Psychiatry, Mount Sinai School of Medicine, City University of New York

ARNOLD WINSTON, M.D.
Director, Department of Psychiatry, Beth Israel Medical Center; and Professor of Clinical Psychiatry, Mount Sinai School of Medicine, City University of New York

Introduction

The material for this monograph developed from a symposium on short-term dynamic psychotherapy (STDP) presented at the American Psychiatric Association meeting in May, 1984. The authors of this monograph have been working together in the Center for Teaching and Research in Short-Term Dynamic Psychotherapy at Beth Israel Medical Center in New York. Our goal has been to develop clinical, teaching, and research programs in short-term dynamic psychotherapy.

The clinical approach of the Center is based on much of the recent work in short-term dynamic psychotherapy. The clinical observations and psychotherapeutic techniques developed by Davanloo (1), Sifneos (2), and Malan (3) have had a major influence on our approach.

We are now using two forms of brief psychotherapy. The first of these is short-term dynamic psychotherapy, and is essentially based on Davanloo's model. This approach focuses primarily on conflict, using psychoanalytic theory as its foundation. Technically, the therapist intervenes whenever resistance appears. The defenses are repeatedly confronted and interpreted, which usually produces a rise in the transference accompanied by a great deal of affect. The transference is actively interpreted, and is linked to current and past persons in the patient's life. In this technique, the focus is maintained; the patient is not allowed to intellectualize or to remain vague.

The second type of short-term psychotherapy is called brief adaptation-oriented psychotherapy (BAP). It is a combination of the Sifneos approach, psychoanalytic psychotherapy, ego psychology, and some cognitive techniques. In this form of psychotherapy, a clear focus is maintained by identifying maladaptive patterns in the patient's behavior. Here, too, resistances are confronted and interpreted. However, the therapist does not relentlessly pursue the resistance. In the same way, transference is not focused upon unless it becomes a clear resistance. This therapy is much more cognitive than is short-term dynamic psychotherapy, which concentrates a great deal on affect.

Both types of therapy aim, as does long-term insight-oriented psychotherapy, not only at symptom remission, but at personality change. All patients are extensively evaluated through the use of standardized instruments and clinical interviews. The evaluation interview usually lasts from two to four hours. The maximum number of sessions is 40; patients are seen once a week. All sessions, including the evaluation interview, are videotaped.

The patients studied at the Center have been those with personality disorders of the histrionic, avoidant, dependent, compulsive, passive-aggressive, and mixed types. Most of the patients also have *DSM-III* Axis I diagnosis, such as generalized anxiety, panic disorder, phobic disorder, dysthymic disorder, and so forth.

In Chapter One, Dr. Been and Ms. Sklar describe short-term dynamic psychotherapy, and point out the importance of the transference in this type of treatment. They describe various transference paradigms, and compare the theoretical and technical differences between short-term dynamic psychotherapy and more traditional analytic psychotherapy.

In Chapter Two, Dr. Goldin and I examine the concept and frequent occurrence of pathological mourning. The techniques used to enable the patient to go through the mourning process are illustrated.

In Chapter Three, Drs. Pollack and Horner discuss the theoretical foundations and the technique of brief adaptation-oriented psychotherapy. Techniques are illustrated with actual patient interviews or clinical vignettes in this, as well as in other, chapters.

In Chapter Four, "The Impact of Short-Term Dynamic Psychotherapy on Psychoanalytic Psychotherapy," Dr. Goldin and I stress the importance of the use of the transference in all psychoanalytic psychotherapy, and note that it is all too often neglected.

Chapter Five, by Drs. Trujillo and McCullough, and Chapter Six, by Dr. Pinsker and associates, present data concerning the patient population and those who have applied for treatment. Drs. Trujillo and McCullough describe pilot data comparing process and outcome in the two types of brief psychotherapy.

It is not our intention to provide a comprehensive review of short-term dynamic psychotherapy within the scope of this monograph. Instead, we attempt to highlight a number of important clinical and research issues in brief psychotherapy.

Arnold Winston, M.D.

References

1. Davanloo H: Techniques of short-term dynamic psychotherapy. Psychiatr Clin North Am 2:11-22, 1979

2. Sifneos P: Short-Term Dynamic Psychotherapy. New York, Plenum Medical Book Company, 1979

3. Malan D: The Frontier of Brief Psychotherapy. New York, Plenum Medical Book Company, 1976

4. Diagnostic and Statistical Manual of Mental Disorders (Third Edition). Washington, D.C., American Psychiatric Association, 1980

1

Transference in Short-Term Dynamic Psychotherapy

Harold Been, M.D.
Isabel Sklar, C.S.W.

1

Transference in Short-Term Dynamic Psychotherapy

The recognition, understanding, and handling of the transference in all dynamic psychotherapies of any duration (from one session to extended psychoanalysis) is central to the unfolding of the clinical interaction and the eventual outcome of the psychotherapy.

In this chapter, the transference phenomena occurring in short-term dynamic psychotherapy will be discussed. The model of short-term psychotherapy, based on principles developed by Dr. Habib Davanloo (1-3), is a highly interpretative, uncovering, and multifocal form of psychotherapy. This therapy is conducted in face-to-face, weekly, 50-minute sessions for as few as six to eight sessions, to as many as 40 sessions. Patients selected for this treatment fall into the neurotic category, and include patients with long-standing characterological problems resistant to other forms of psychotherapy. Before discussing the specific transference phenomena occurring in short-term dynamic psychotherapy, the concept of transference used in this chapter will be discussed. This will be followed by a comparison of the technical requirements of short-term dynamic psychotherapy with those of classical psychoanalysis.

DEFINITION OF TRANSFERENCE

The concept of transference used in this chapter encompasses all the feelings, fantasies, and reactions, conscious or unconscious, experienced by the patient toward the therapist. These feelings, thoughts, and reactions are stimulated by the real relationship between the patient and therapist, the patient's characterological style, and classic transference potentialities. The classic definition of the transference, defined by Greenson (4), is the "experiencing of feelings, drives, attitudes, fantasies, and defenses toward a person in the present which do not befit that person, but are a repetition of reactions originating in regard to significant persons of childhood, unconsciously displaced onto figures in the present" (p. 155). Gill (5) has commented upon the various stimuli affecting the patient in the therapeutic process, and argues that the stimuli are all interwoven. He argues that the therapist should always examine the underlying, unconscious transference meaning in the patient's productions in a therapeutic hour, regardless of the real stimuli influencing the patient. This, however, requires that the therapist be aware of the process variables he or she is or is not using (that is, activity versus passivity) in the therapeutic setting. It is otherwise impossible to properly assess and empathize with the patient's reactions. The forceful, overt presence of a therapist using the more focused techniques found in short-term psychotherapies has, in itself, a major transference impact. Thus, process variables and content variables within any therapeutic interaction are always intimately related and mutually dependent upon each other.

COMPARISON OF TECHNIQUES IN CLASSICAL ANALYSIS VERSUS SHORT-TERM DYNAMIC PSYCHOTHERAPY

The techniques used in classical analysis and in short-term dynamic psychotherapy have strong similarities. They both use techniques of clarification, confrontation, interpretation, and working through. Both use the transference as a pivotal tool in engaging the patient and in working through the conflicts. Both techniques seek to reach into the patient's internal world by using fantasy material and dreams as meaningful reflections of the patient's unconscious. A fundamental difference between classical analysis and short-term dynamic psychotherapy stems from the way the transference is used to engage the patient in a profound emotional experience, linking the current emotional experiences with those of early life.

In classical analysis, the central tool is the development and resolution of the transference neurosis. The term transference neurosis as defined by Greenson (4) "describes that constellation of transference reactions in which the analyst and the analysis have become the center of the patient's neurotic conflicts relived in the analytic situation" (p. 34). Freud (6-9) concluded that the only way to unlock the core infantile neurosis was to allow the patient to fully relive the infantile conflicts and later derivatives in relation to the analyst by way of the transference neurosis. The repetitive working through of the experiences with the analyst provides the leverage to bring about change. Thus, psychoanalytic techniques are designed to promote the development of the transference neurosis without interference. The necessary regression in the service of the ego is promoted by a neutral, relatively nonintrusive stance, in which the patient's free associations lead the analytic inquiry until resistances occur.

The conscious therapeutic alliance involving the patient's observing ego is sensitively and gently fostered by the gradual interpretation of derivative material: those productions that unconsciously use specific interpersonal situations to disguise other interpersonal contexts. The use of derivatives often serves the patient's unconscious need to maintain distance in the transference. In psychoanalysis, derivative material is not systematically challenged during the day-to-day work. Interpretations linking past, present, and transference figures are only made when the patient, through his productions, shows overt readiness for them. The technical requirements of this process necessitate frequent weekly visits over an extended period of time. Technical difficulties arise secondary to the tenacity of the regressive, dependent, and passive yearnings inherent in the development of the transference neurosis. A lengthy analysis is often required to handle the resolution of the more symbiotic features. It is questionable if these issues are ever completely resolved.

In contrast, the initial goal in short-term dynamic psychotherapy is to immediately promote the development of the unconscious therapeutic alliance. This is defined as the patient's spontaneous production of material deriving from unconscious, internalized object relationships. This material emerges through the adaptive context of a session or through dreams or fresh memories. As abundant psychoanalytic work has demonstrated, this material can only be obtained when the characterological armor, as defined by Reich (10), is meaningfully punctured. "If one neglects such character resistances, and instead simply follows the line of the material, such resistances form a ballast which it is difficult, if not impossible, to remove. One gains more and more the impression that every interpretation of meaning was wasted, that the patient continues to doubt everything, or only pretends to accept things, or that he meets everything with an inward smile. If the elimination of these resistances was not begun right in the beginning, they confront one with an insuperable obstacle in the later stages of analysis" (p. 51). Patients in psychosocial crises also demonstrate the availability of such unconscious material because their defensive structures have been loosened by the crises. It has also been clinically evident that the experience of intense affect in psychotherapy sessions is followed by meaningful early unconscious material.

Davanloo (1, 2) emphasizes that a crisis, if not already present, needs to be created for the patient in each and every session by actively pushing at the patient's characterological defenses or psychodynamic resistances immediately as they occur. Characterological resistances not systematically addressed in psychoanalysis, such as language, body posture, and so forth, are vigorously challenged, thus creating the crisis for the patient in the here and now with the therapist. A careful monitoring of the patient's defensive structure and level of anxiety protects the process from undermining a fragile ego structure. For further details of technique the reader is referred to the technical writings of Davanloo (1, 2).

In short-term dynamic psychotherapy, the living experience in the transference is the central tool of the psychotherapy. The living experience encompasses the following:

1. All defenses against emotional experience in a specific interpersonal context: that is, obsessional and hysterical defenses are vigorously clarified, confronted, and interpreted early in the therapy, until the underlying affect is explicitly experienced with both cognitive and physiological components.
2. Regressive tendencies experienced in the transference: that is, helplessness, dependency, and passivity are immediately challenged, as are similar defenses against genuine affectual experience.
3. Any sign of resistance to clear communication without affective resonance is immediately challenged. As treatment progresses, the affectual intensity need not always be at a maximal level.
4. The patient is always reminded and encouraged to work in the treatment using his ego capacities to the fullest. For instance, patients are often reminded of their capacity to undermine and defeat the therapist by the use of regressive defenses. This places the responsibility for the therapy with the patient.

The constant interpretation of the patient's regression and his resistance to communicate clearly with the therapist prevents the repetitive communication of derivative material and the subsequent development of the transference neurosis. The repeated experience of strong affects after analysis of the characterological defenses forms one of the major focuses of the working-through process. This procedure also serves to desensitize the patient's ego to otherwise toxic affects.

Another technical requirement in short-term dynamic psychotherapy is the active focusing of the treatment, rather than the strict use of the patient's free associations. The core genetic conflict underlying the patient's current areas of disturbance are delineated in a comprehensive evaluation prior to the onset of treatment. During the therapy, the therapist actively maintains the focus on the resistances or on the adaptive context. The adaptive context is defined as the most salient current manifestation of the patient's core difficulties as evidenced by the patient's verbal and nonverbal communication. Throughout the course of the therapy, the therapist maintains the focus on issues related to the core problems.

The techniques used to avoid the transference neurosis and regression, and to focus the interaction, promote repeated intense therapist-patient interactions in a highly charged atmosphere. The patient's mixed feelings toward the therapist are explored and connected immediately to similar feelings experienced with current and past figures. This results in a working-through process of repeated transference–current figure–past figure linkages (TCP interpretations), which prevents lingering in the transference. Malan (11, 12) has shown that the frequency of TCP linkages has a very high correlation with a positive outcome in dynamic psychotherapy.

The proper application of technique results in the patient's reliving the early genetic experiences with full intensity, yet with minimal regression, in contrast to reliving the early experiences through the emotional storms of the transference neurosis. The absence of the transference neurosis also prevents the protracted termination phase characteristic of classical analysis.

TRANSFERENCE PARADIGMS IN SHORT-TERM DYNAMIC PSYCHOTHERAPY

In short-term dynamic psychotherapy, the therapist's first goal, as stated earlier, is to quickly challenge the patient's characterological resistances. This is accomplished by a systematic analysis of the characterological defenses. The patient always responds to this with anxiety and further neurotic defenses designed to prevent the therapist from entering his inner world. The patient also responds with intense ambivalence: longing for closeness with a strong therapist to help fight the neurotic structure, as well as experiencing the therapist as an intruder into the familiarity of his inner world. This resonates with the early ambivalence toward the original primary figures: that is, fear of an intrusive, controlling father, versus a wish for a nonpassive father; fear of a castrating mother, versus a wish for a strong, caring mother; and so forth. The constant implicit appeal to the patient's ego to allow the therapist into his inner life is the driving force behind the therapeutic interaction. By not allowing the patient to regress, and by placing the responsibility for the work onto the patient, both the conscious and unconscious therapeutic alliances are enhanced during this process.

The therapist's active intrusion into the patient's inner world stimulates resistances that are often explicitly manifest as a negative transference or a regressive defense. In short-term dynamic psychotherapy, as opposed to classical analysis, the rapid stimulation and analysis of the aggressive impulses and accompanying regressive defenses predominates in the early phase of the therapy, particularly in patients with obsessive character structures.

Very often, in many obsessional characters, the superego is very harsh and primitive. The underlying sadistic impulses promote masochistic defenses. These defenses defeat the therapist and the patient. They are often manifest in negative therapeutic reactions that result in abrupt termination. Thus, with obsessive characters, the first task is to rapidly challenge the defenses blocking the sadistic impulses. This alleviates the superego's hold on the therapeutic process. As the therapist confronts the patient's character structure, the patient defends against the intrusion until there is a breakthrough of the underlying hostile impulses. Often these impulses are expressed toward the therapist. Repetitive desensitization of the ego to these impulses frees the patient to experience the underlying libidinal impulses. This is often accompanied by the derepression of earlier memories.

The following clinical vignette illustrates the transference phenomena previously described:

> The patient is a 35-year-old, obsessional, married man with a masochistic character structure surrounding intense repressed hostile

> impulses. The beginning sessions focused on the hostility experienced toward his wife and professional colleagues. In the sixth session, the focus shifted to his feelings toward his mother. In the eighth session, the patient verbalized anger with his mother, who had just celebrated her 75th birthday. He was angry at her for expressing indifferent feelings toward a 90-year-old male family friend who had been very helpful to her.

The patient stated he was angry, but he was unable to describe his experience of anger. Instead, what emerged were obsessional defenses. The patient's defenses were repetitively challenged, and were accompanied by repeated questioning of his inner experience of the anger. (The inner experience of a feeling encompasses the motoric, physiologic, cognitive, and fantasy components accompanying a stated feeling.) The patient was clearly resistant and continued to defend against the underlying murderous rage with passivity, vagueness, and helplessness. As his regressive stance was continually challenged, the patient's voice became louder and his physical movements became more active. It was clear that the patient was experiencing motoric evidence of affect. Further challenging his use of helplessness produced a continued rise in the patient's affect. At this point the therapist made the patient explicitly aware of his affect, and the patient was again asked to describe his inner experience of anger toward the therapist. After clarifying the use of obsessional defenses against the anger in the transference, the therapist again returned to explore the anger toward the patient's mother.

Up to this point in the session, the therapist extensively confronted the patient's characterological defenses against the experience of his feelings. Without this confrontation, the patient's communications were flat and relatively uninformative. This confrontation produced anger toward the therapist, a frequent occurrence in this type of treatment. A significant crisis was introduced into the session, loosening the patient's defensive structure. The patient was experiencing, in the here and now, his buried rage toward the therapist and the struggle to contain that feeling. With the breakthrough of intense affect, the subsequent material had significant dynamic meaning.

> The patient again described the scene at his mother's birthday party, but with greater feeling. He remembered that he "froze for a second" at the moment of his fury toward his mother. He described an image of lashing out and striking his mother under her chin with severe force. The patient acknowledged that his mother would have been severely hurt or even killed by the force of his blow. Tears filled his eyes as he described the fantasy of the murder and its consequence: the loss of his mother, for whom he also had tender feelings. With this communication, the patient was deeply immersed in profound ambivalent feelings toward his mother. He was obviously moved and completely taken with this living experience with the therapist.
>
> In the following session, the patient spoke of his thoughts about the preceding session. The patient recalled an early set of memories during the previous week. In early latency, he had been given two teddy bears by his two older sisters. He recalled that every night he would alternately hug them and make them engage in very violent fights. Eventually the head was knocked off of one of the teddy bears. This memory contained the childhood expression of his mixed feelings—his sadism and his tenderness. The early family context of his powerful ambivalent feelings was then ripe for exploration. This recollection also reflected a strong unconscious therapeutic alliance that was stimulated in the previous session. This type of progression and result is typical of the process in every session.

The unconscious sources of these negative feelings in the transference stem from multiple intrapsychic forces other than the overt resistance to characterological challenge produced by the technique. The sources of the negative transference stem from id, ego, and superego resistances, as they do in classical analysis. However, the manifestations in short-term dynamic psychotherapy are heightened by the patient's intense intrapsychic experience of intrusion.

The superego resistances are stimulated by the patient's unconscious perception that if the therapist is allowed to enter into the patient's inner life, the therapist will become closer to the patient than the patient has permitted any earlier objects to become. In obsessional patients such as the one described, one or many early objects—mother, father, siblings, and so on—are experienced with intense murderous rage by the patient. The patient subsequently distanced himself from them in order to avoid the consequences of this rage: murder, loss, and retaliation. This resulted in distant relationships and unconscious guilt. The patient's realization of the wish for closeness with the therapist presents him with a severe conflict. He must protect himself from the resurgence of these murderous impulses and remain loyal in a masochistic surrender to the punished early objects. This superego resistance repeatedly appears as the patient further allows the therapist into his inner life. Thus, in the previous clinical vignette, it is not only the active intrusion into the patient's characterological armor that triggers resistance. By allowing the therapist to know his intimate feelings—in this case, murderous—the patient's intrapsychic economy is threatened.

The id resistances are stimulated by the patient's unconscious perception that if the therapist is permitted to get close to the patient's emotional life, this will threaten the libidinal attachment to early objects and eventually displace them. The result would be movement toward the depressive position, which the patient defensively avoids. This resistance is present in every patient, but is particularly powerful in those who have had an intense attachment to one parent. This attachment was heightened by an early illness in the patient, or by an early loss of the other parent through death, separation, or experienced rejection. Frequently, the therapist's threat to the early libidinal attachment is also experienced unconsciously as an intrusive oedipal and/or sibling rival, depending upon the patient's history.

The following clinical example illustrates this resistance:

> The patient, a middle aged, divorced mother of two children, sought treatment for her current difficulties with men. She lost her father when she was eight or nine years old, and had never been able to mourn this loss despite many years of psychotherapy. After the first ten minutes of the evaluation, the therapist commented that the patient frequently averted her eyes. The patient became noticeably anxious, and asked if the therapy required her to look into the therapist's eyes. The therapist asked what she felt when she looked at the therapist. With obvious anxiety and in a shaky voice, the patient tried to express what she felt. Initially, she described what she saw, but the therapist again asked her what she experienced. Tears came to her

eyes and she tried to look away. A reminder to the patient of her turning her eyes away from the therapist produced more forceful tears; she then expressed deep sadness.

In this initial contact, the therapist focused on the distancing defenses the patient used to avoid meaningful human contact despite her ease in verbal conversation. Though it was obvious that there was sadness and grief behind her distancing maneuvers, the full significance of this was yet to be understood.

Later in the interview, the patient was asked to describe her father. As she began to speak, she broke into tears. She could only remember the back of his head. Further exploration of early memories of the father were accompanied by anxiety and tears. Here, again, the deeper significance of the patient's earlier distancing maneuvers in the transference became more evident. She was desperately trying to keep her feelings about her father repressed and undisturbed. Obviously, anyone who attempted to get close to her would be faced with exclusion in order to keep the early fantasies stable within the unconscious and avoid the painful experience of loss. The therapist's eyes were both a link to the memory of her father's eyes and a threatened displacement of those memories. The treatment of this woman would require constant confrontation of her distancing defenses in the transference and in her current life. These repeated transference confrontations would be necessary in order to aid the derepression of the earlier memories and fantasies of her father.

The ego resistances stem from a patient's unconscious perception that if the therapist is permitted to enter the patient's inner life, the closeness will result in a severe loss: that is, death. This is true with patients who have actually experienced the loss of a parent or other important figures. This was true with the female patient in the previous case example, whose fear of closeness with the therapist was also linked with death due to her early loss.

Besides the id, ego, and superego resistances stimulated by the intrusion of the therapist, the more classic transference reactions also occur and result in resistances. The transference of feelings from early figures onto the therapist occurs regularly: that is, the mother or father transference. These are immediately clarified, interpreted, and worked through during the course of each session. For patients who have lost important figures in their early lives, pathological or unfinished mourning must be reawakened and worked through. In short-term dynamic psychotherapy, pathological mourning needs to be addressed early in the treatment. This is crucial because the defensive structure surrounding the unfinished mourning freezes the entire character structure. Significant change cannot occur until this is resolved. Further elaboration of pathological mourning is found elsewhere in this monograph.

Underneath the negative transference, the powerful longing for closeness always emerges and is intensely experienced in short-term dynamic psychotherapy. Genuine erotic and passive longings and fantasies occur in the mid-phase of treatment. It should be noted that the early appearance of erotic longings in the transference is defensive, and is interpreted as such. The full erotic transference seen in the transference neurosis with its regressive and aggressive underpinnings is avoided in short-term dynamic psychotherapy, because the characterological defenses and the negative transference have been systematically analyzed. The structured transference constellations of penis envy in women and passive homosexuality in men are also avoided for similar reasons. The libidinal components associated with the erotic transference, penis envy, and male passive homosexuality do occur, but they are readily accessible to analysis.

Typically, the transference paradigms unfold as follows: initial characterological work; analysis of pathological mourning, if present; repeated analyses of the negative transference and accompanying resistance; deepening of the unconscious therapeutic alliance; analysis of the genuine erotic and passive yearnings with the accompanying defenses against closeness; and a brief analysis of the separation from the therapist in the final phase.

The termination phase is not usually dramatic, and is either initiated by the patient or by the therapist. The reason for this is that the preceding analysis has dealt with loss early in the treatment while avoiding the transference neurosis. In patients who have experienced an actual early loss, the final phase is characterized by the working through of the patient's experience of loss in the transference, and by the linking of the loss with remaining unanalyzed earlier losses. This is not a protracted process, and may take between three and five sessions.

Though patients experience intense struggle and anxiety while undergoing short-term dynamic psychotherapy, they also experience gratitude and relief throughout the treatment. They long for genuine closeness with another human being. As the therapist refuses to accept the neurotic need for distancing and emotional isolation, patients experience a growing sense of intimacy. A proper holding environment a la Winnicott (13) is provided.

Discussion

Psychodynamic psychotherapy has certain implicit assumptions derived from its psychoanalytic underpinnings. The work currently being done in short-term dynamic psychotherapy provides impetus for questioning these basic assumptions. The assumptions relating to transference are as follows:

1. Regression in the transference over a period of time is required to reach and work through in-depth material systematically.
2. The experience and analysis of all the regressive yearnings and fantasies implicit in the unfolding of the transference neurosis are fundamental to the reconstruction of character structure.
3. In order to assure noncontamination of the transference and to avoid suggestion, the therapist should assume a nonintrusive posture.

The uncovering of fresh, early memories and fantasy parallels changes in personality and in fantasy structure regularly in short-term dynamic psychotherapy patients. Long-term followup by Davanloo suggests these changes are permanent and structural, not a transference cure. The above findings require further systematic research and clinical investigation.

Freud's genius unlocked the language of the unconscious for clinical study. He also made possible the study of interpersonal process variables through his discovery of transference phenomena. The work of Reich, as mentioned earlier, emphasized the clinical need for a breach in the ego syntonic characterological defensive structure in order to effect a meaningful analysis of unconscious material. The later work of the interpersonal school—such as the work of Sullivan (14) and the communication analysts such as Haley (15)—shed further light on the nature and importance of process variables in understanding dyadic relationships. They demonstrated that paradoxical communications immediately helped to breach the defensive structure of patients, thus producing a heightened intensity of exchange. There has been a gradual theoretical and clinical fusion of Freud's and Reich's early discoveries with the later understanding of process variables in most modern psychoanalytic thinking.

Clinically, however, analytic therapists, whatever their theoretical biases, avoid the systematic, active use of process variables because they are thought to be too intrusive. Therapists patiently await their cues from the patient's verbal productions in timing their interpretations. The primary concern is the respect for the patient's defenses, the preservation of autonomy, and the avoidance of stimulating excessive anxiety. These concerns are critical but all too often offer a rationale for passivity. It is clear from the work in short-term dynamic psychotherapy that accepting free associations and derivative material is often an unwitting collusion with the patient's defensive need to avoid current, meaningful communication in the transference.

The masochistic male patient described earlier was warding off his sadistic feelings and the anxiety that would accompany the breakthrough of impulses with intense unconscious genetic meaning. He was unconsciously appealing to the therapist to be strong enough to accept these impulses in order to master them, and at the same time fighting the therapist's challenge in order to remain loyal to his past objects. The therapist could have accepted the patient's helplessness as a genuine message that his underlying anxiety was too strong. The resultant regression would have alleviated both the patient's anxiety and the therapist's fear of an intense affectual exchange.

Similarly, the previously discussed female patient's warding off of her grief through distancing was an unconscious appeal for the therapist's acceptance of the full intensity of her genuine grief. For the therapist to not continue the full challenge of her neurotic, emotional isolation, as manifested in the aversion of her eyes, would also have been to collude with her regressive tendencies. Again, the therapist's potential anxiety in the face of powerful affects could have diverted the therapeutic process into less anxious channels. It is Davanloo's particular genius to read the patient's moment to moment defensive communications (the characterological defenses) as immediate attempts to ward off the patient's current wish for the therapist's intrusion into his inner world. Thus, the paradoxical situation of the therapist's persistent, systematic challenging of the defenses creates a powerful breach in these defenses, enabling the therapist to rapidly engage with the patient's deepest ambivalent longings for genuine closeness with the original objects.

SUMMARY

The evolving transferential process in short-term dynamic psychotherapy resulting from changes in analytic technique discussed in this chapter emphasizes the need for the continuing study of process variables and their relationship to content variables and potential transference paradigms. The understanding of these interrelationships and the resulting clinical outcomes await further research. Only in this manner will psychodynamic psychotherapy evolve into a more efficient process and toward a more scientific position. The understanding of these interrelationships will also lead to the rethinking of basic metapsychological concepts, thus enriching the current body of psychoanalytic thought.

References

1. Davanloo H: Principles and Techniques of Short-Term Dynamic Psychotherapy. New York, Spectrum Press, 1978

2. Davanloo H: Techniques of Short-Term Dynamic Psychotherapy. Psychiatr Clin North Am 2(1):11-22, 1979

3. Davanloo H: Short-Term Dynamic Psychotherapy. New York, Jason Aronson, 1980

4. Greenson RR: The Technique and Practice of Psychoanalysis. New York, International Universities Press, 1967

5. Gill M: Analysis of Transference, vol. I. New York, International Universities Press, 1982

6. Freud S: The dynamics of transference 1912, in Complete Psychological Works, Standard Edition, vol. 12. Translated and edited by Strachey J. London, Hogarth Press, 1955

7. Freud S: Observations on transference-love, further recommendations on the technique of psychoanalysis III (1915), in Complete Psychological Works, Standard Edition, vol. 12. Translated and edited by Strachey J. London, Hogarth Press, 1955

8. Freud S: On beginning treatment: further recommendations on the technique of psychoanalysis (1913), in Complete Psychological Works, Standard Edition, vol. 12. Translated and edited by Strachey J. London, Hogarth Press, 1955

9. Freud S: Remembering, repeating and working-through (1914), in Complete Psychological Works, Standard Edition, vol. 12. London, Hogarth Press, 1955

10. Reich W: Character Analysis. New York, Noonday Press, 1949

11. Malan DH: Toward the Validation of Dynamic Psychotherapy. New York, Plenum Medical Books, 1976

12. Malan DH: Individual Psychotherapy and the Science of Psychodynamics. London, Butterworths, 1979

13. Winnicott DW: The Maturational Processes and the Facilitating Environment. New York, International Universities Press, 1965

14. Sullivan HS: Clinical Studies in Psychiatry. Edited by Perry HS,

Gawel ML, Gibbons M. New York, W.W. Norton and Company, 1956

15. Haley J: Strategies of Psychotherapy. New York, Grune and Stratton, 1963

2

Pathological Mourning in Short-Term Dynamic Psychotherapy

Arnold Winston, M.D.
Victor Goldin, M.D.

2

Pathological Mourning in Short-Term Dynamic Psychotherapy

Pathological mourning is a frequently overlooked but important psychiatric condition. Early recognition and skillful exploration of this problem adds clarity to the psychotherapeutic process and leads to a more positive, stable outcome (1). Davanloo (2) calls attention to the importance of pathological mourning in crisis resolution. He has also commented on pathological mourning as a significant factor in short-term dynamic psychotherapy (personal communication).

Early psychoanalytic writers (3, 4) laid the groundwork for the appreciation of pathological mourning. Lindemann (5) refocused attention on acute and delayed grief and pathological and normal mourning. Bowlby (6), describing loss in children, further expanded this field.

Despite work done by these and other authors, however, the critical importance of pathological mourning still often goes unrecognized. This is unfortunate, since in our recent clinical experience, almost one-half of a large number of patients evaluated in our Center had significant evidence of pathological mourning (7). It is our thesis that short-term dynamic psychotherapy is a technique uniquely suited to resolve this condition.

In this chapter we focus on the real, as opposed to symbolic, loss through death of a significant person. We are adopting this narrow view for the sake of clarity. While there is something similar in the loss of a desired oedipal object to a rival (8), the loss and mourning of the separation-individuation phase (9), or in the loss of a best friend who moves 1,000 miles away, we feel that our purpose is best served by building from a base on which the most concrete and easily discernible cases are clarified.

Having limited the territory to be explored, let us turn to some basic definitions. It is unfortunate that there is no agreed upon meaning for the key words, mourning and grief. We will follow the definition used by the Langley Porter group (10). In this chapter, "grief refers to the phenomena of subjective experience and behavior that occurs after a loss. Normal or successful mourning refers to processes in which states of grief are eventually attenuated with the adapatation to loss. Pathological grief is the intensification of grief to the level where the person is overwhelmed, resorts to maladaptive behavior, or remains interminably in a state of grief without progression of the mourning process toward completion. Pathological mourning involves processes that do not move progressively toward assimilation or accomodation, but instead lead to stereotyped repetitions or extensive interruptions of healing" (p. 1157).

We wish to emphasize our basic belief throughout this chapter that when pathological mourning is the outcome of loss, the potential effect on the person involved is always significant.

Brown and Stoudemire (11), building on the seminal work of Lindemann, have divided mourning into approximately three distinct phases. The first phase is characterized by "a state of shock or numbed disbelief" (p. 378). Lindemann describes "sensations of somatic distress occurring in waves lasting from 20 minutes to an hour at a time, the feeling of tightness in the throat, choking with shortness of breath, need for sighing and an empty feeling in the abdomen, lack of muscular power, and an intense subjective distress described as tension or mental pain" (p. 141). Brown and Stoudemire add that "patients may feel lost, dazed, stunned, helpless, immobilized, and disorganized" (p. 378). Characteristically, this phase lasts from one to 14 days.

In normal mourning, the numbness quickly gives way to

experiencing painful sadness of the loss. It is during this phase that somatic symptoms, anorexia, insomnia, fatigue, and weakness appear. Crying spells may persist, and the aggrieved becomes preoccupied with memories of the deceased. This includes recalling the past relationship in great detail. The survivor may feel guilty and angry toward the lost person.

The return to normal interests and the recall of past relationships with the deceased, now sometimes colored with pleasant memories, indicates movement toward the resolution phase. Brown and Stoudemire note that "crying spells, feelings of emptiness and the longing for the dead still occur, but tend to diminish in intensity and duration" (p. 379). Normal mourning may persist for six months to one year. However, "symptoms" may be activated on an anniversary of the death or on special occasions.

The clinician needs to be aware of these indicators of normal mourning as he or she examines the reaction to the loss of important objects. Detailed inquiry into these processes is necessary to differentiate normal from pathological mourning. Because patients are often separated from the event by many years, the interviewer must utilize a highly focused approach that enables the patient to recall significant details.

Case Example "A"

A 45-year-old businessman presented to the Center for Short-Term Dynamic Psychotherapy with suicidal ideas, depression, and anxiety. Some of his distress was related to repeated job failures associated with conflicts with authority. He spoke of his wife of ten years as "critical and nonsupportive." The patient had several previous episodes of depression, the most serious of which occurred during college, and which resulted in hospitalization.

The patient's childhood was brought to an abrupt close when his father, a prominent businessman ("tall, handsome, admired by all") died of a massive heart attack. The patient, then 14, came home from school on an ordinary spring afternoon. He found his home filled with strangers. He went upstairs to change his clothes. His mother followed him and told him that his father had died. The achievement of his father's admiration had been the elusive goal of his earlier years. He was stunned and confused. He cried only once during the funeral week.

In the months following his father's death, he was the frequent victim of attacks by his peers. His provocative behavior led to severe beatings. Three years later, in college, he would first excel in courses and then fail to complete papers and final examinations. This self-defeating behavior continued in his business career. Now, 31 years later, he could recall little about the week his father died and the weeks that followed, despite repeated efforts by the interviewer to focus on the details.

During the third psychotherapy session, the therapist continued to focus on the father's death and ask detailed questions. Again the patient responded blandly, "I don't remember any more about that week." This vagueness was repeatedly challenged. The therapist noticed that the patient began to squirm and smile. These subtle nonverbal responses were pointed out. This was met first with denial and then with a gradually developing hostility. The anger toward the therapist was interpreted. As this affect was more fully experienced, it led to a new set of memories. At this point, the patient smiled again and recalled with some embarrassment: "This is hard, I'm surprised. I haven't thought about this in years. I was looking at my father in the coffin, and I suddenly thought of a joke about a man with a terrific tan who died. The punch line was he never looked better in his life. I smiled then, I had to try hard to keep from laughing. I sweated and squirmed a bit. I felt . . . how could I laugh at my father's funeral?"

This recollection unblocked an outpouring of details about his father and his father's death. These were accompanied by increasingly vivid affect. As the negative connotations of the "chapel humor" scene were explored, the latent angry feelings toward the father developed more fully. This, in turn, was followed by an avalanche of sobbing . . . with positive, tender feelings for his father. The exposed ambivalence was worked with extensively in subsequent sessions.

In this case example, the therapist recognized the necessity of focusing on the patient's pathological grief. When the patient is seen many years after the loss, it is usually more difficult to elicit details surrounding the death, and even harder to reach the associated affect.

The therapist pursued and focused on detailed descriptions of the father's death and funeral. The patient resisted with vagueness that was challenged. The nonverbal responses of the patient were pointed out, and anger toward the therapist emerged in a veiled manner. The anger was interpreted, and led to the memory of the joke. The joke brought with it an outpouring of feelings and memories concerning the father.

The unresolved mourning proved to be closely linked to pathological behavior that colored his life from that point on. While his maladaptive behavior had additional roots, the pathological mourning was a major contributor to his life-long failures. In this case, the therapist might have focused his or her attention on the marital difficulty or on the conflicts at work. However, the initial evaluation revealed the presence of pathological mourning. Thus, forewarned, the therapist was alerted to thoroughly explore this area.

The concept of pathological mourning can be traced to Freud (3) and Abraham (4). Freud found that ambivalence toward the lost object is often present before the loss. Once the loss takes place, identification with the lost object occurs, followed by aggression against the object. Freud stated "the shadow of the object fell upon the ego." The anger originally felt toward the object is then directed at the internalized lost object; that is, the self.

Freud attempted to distinguish normal mourning from pathological mourning (melancholia) noting that in normal mourning the rage and aggression toward the object is not present. Subsequent authors, such as Lindemann (5), Bowlby (6), and Joffe and Sandler (12) have not found this distinction to be clinically accurate. Persons going through normal mourning can also have feelings of hostility and anger. Joffe and Sandler explain the aggression toward the lost object as deriving from frustrated wishes and longing for that which is lost. The mourner turns his aggression against the source of pain. If excessive aggression persists, the mourner may develop pathological mourning. When there is excessive anger and aggression toward the lost object, guilt becomes a major issue. The greater the ambivalence and rage, the more important the guilt becomes (2, 3, 13, 14).

In 1944, Lindemann (5) reported on acute grief, based in large part on his experience with survivors of the Coconut Grove fire in Boston. Lindemann showed that acute grief may appear after a crisis, may be delayed or exaggerated, or at times may be apparently absent. We are focusing on a group of patients in whom the acute grief appears to be absent.

Bowlby (6) found that many patients with pathological mourning had a loss of a parent in childhood. He described four types of pathological mourning due to loss: "*1.* persistent and unconscious yearning to recover the lost object; *2.* anger and reproach to various objects, including the self; *3.* caring for someone else who has also been bereaved; *4.* denial that the object is permanently lost" (pp. 501-502). These four types of pathological mourning often occur in combination and do not fall into mutually exclusive categories. Bowlby felt that of the four, yearning for the lost object was the most prevalent and important type of pathologic response.

Helene Deutsch (15) described an adult with a "wooden and affectionless character" whose mother died when he was five years old. In this case, as an adult, the patient expressed only negative and aggressive attitudes toward his mother.

As one looks at the work of Freud, Lindemann, Bowlby, Joffe and Sandler, Deutsch, and others, two major themes become clear. One theme is a libidinal attachment and yearning for the lost object; the other theme is the presence of aggressive and angry impulses toward the object. These ambivalent feelings often are related to positive and negative past experiences that the patient has had with the lost object and with other important persons. Ferenczi (16) felt that such ambivalence is developmental and arises in early infant-parent interactions, consisting of indulgence or gratification, alternating with deprivation or frustration. When the parent gratifies, positive feelings are produced; when the parent deprives, negative feelings are produced.

Mahler and colleagues (9), in describing sequential stages in normal development, see the relinquishing of the symbiotic bond with mother and moving into the separation-individuation phase as producing a mourning process. Gradually the omnipotent mother is given up and integrated, and discrete positive images of self and object emerge. However, if the mother is either too frustrating or overindulgent, integrated self and object images do not develop, and serious psychopathology may ensue.

Horowitz and colleagues (10) describe negative self and object images being held in check by a given object. With the loss of the object, a shift occurs, and the negative self and object images emerge. Put more simply, if important objects such as a mother or father do not die, the feelings toward object and self are continuously adjusted by real life events.

It is clear, then, that there are a number of important, dynamic considerations in pathological mourning. The first and most obvious dynamic is the loss itself and the resultant shift in the positive and negative self and object representations. If the shift is a marked one, significant developmental difficulties may be present. Severe splitting, a lack of self-object differentiation, and so forth, indicate serious psychopathology of the borderline or narcissistic type. We will focus here on patients whose psychopathology is primarily conflictual rather than developmental. Patients with more severe psychopathology are, in general, not candidates for short-term dynamic psychotherapy.

Another critical issue, as we have mentioned, is the extent and magnitude of the libidinal attachment, versus the aggressive or murderous feelings toward the lost object. The depth and relative mixture of the libidinal and aggressive impulses depend both on the patient's past experiences with the lost object and on the patient's stage of development when the loss occurs. When the aggressive impulses predominate, the conflict with the lost object often continues on an unconscious basis. When the positive feelings prevail, the patient may refuse to give up the lost object. The object is retained and new attachments are blocked. As Freud (3) noted, "It is a matter of general observation that people never willingly abandon a libidinal position" (p. 244). Kohut (17) carries this point further, so that in his formulation aggression has no part. He views the continued libidinal attachment to the lost object as the primary factor in pathological mourning. However, in our view, the libidinal and aggressive impulses are both important, and depend on the patient's psychological development and relationship with the lost object.

When the loss occurs in childhood, the developmental stage of the child is an important determinant of the type of response. For example, a loss during the oedipal stage of the same sex parent presents the child with an oedipal victory. This may lead to the unconscious belief that he or she murdered the parent with the resultant development of profound guilt, and the turning away from the parent of the opposite sex. The type of reaction to a loss in an adult will depend more directly on the personality structure. For example, an obsessional person may react with little affect to a loss; a patient with a hysterical personality may react with much greater affect.

TECHNICAL CONSIDERATIONS

The techniques used to uncover and work through pathological mourning are derived from those generally used in short-term dynamic psychotherapy (18, 19). Patients must be suitable for an approach based on a conflict model and not a developmental one. Short-term dynamic psychotherapy should not be applied to those patients with significant pre-oedipal psychopathology. Case examples will be used to help illustrate the various techniques.

Case Example "B"

A 43-year-old man presented to the Center for short-term dynamic psychotherapy with anxiety, fear of death, and an inability to develop a sustained relationship with a woman.

The patient was the youngest child in a working class family. His early childhood was characterized by a clinging relationship with his mother and an exceedingly ambivalent relationship with his father. After high school he entered the marines and later became a policeman. Physical prowess, fighting, and drinking were highly valued by the patient and by his brothers.

When the patient was in his late 20s, his father died. His mother died ten years later. While in his 30s, he enrolled in college and eventually became an accountant.

He had a number of relationships with women, but all of these ended as soon as the patient perceived that they might develop into something more permanent.

During the evaluation interview, a great deal of anger emerged in relation to the interviewer. This was linked to previously expressed anger toward his boss. The focus then shifted to his older brother, with whom he had a highly ambivalent relationship. From there the interview moved to an exploration of his relationship with his father.

P: And I remember thinking that he might kill her, or punch her and that frightened me, but I used to have fantasies of killing him if he hurt my mother. I remember being in my bedroom upstairs . . .

T: And you were how old?

P: Five, six. They used to have these arguments and I always took the side of my mother, I didn't intellectualize the argument—I just could hear them bellowing.

T: You were in your bed and where were they?

P: Downstairs in the kitchen. I think I would go to my bedroom or if I wasn't there that seemed to be a refuge or something. So I would go there and listen to them having these arguments and they would frighten me. I thought they would split up, because one or two times my mother went to her mother's house, which frightened me. I was very attached to my mother. I mean really crazily attached to my mother. When she would go out at night I would start screaming and crying.

T: When they were battling and you were in your bed, what were you experiencing?

P: Fright and rage and fear because I used to play out this scenario where he would beat up my mother and I would come down and get a kitchen knife and stab him.

T: You would stab him where?

P: In the back. He would like hit on my mother or be over her or something, beating her up and I would stab him in the back. (Patient appears visibly agitated.)

T: Then what would happen? He would be . . .

P: He would be dead.

T: He would be dead.

P: Yes.

T: And then?

P: I didn't carry it that far I don't think. The whole thing just frightened me.

T: But he would be dead and killed and out of the picture—eliminated.

There was further exploration of this fantasy, and the therapist then asked if his feelings toward his father changed.

P: I grew closer to my father. I learned to have very strong feelings toward my father—I learned to sympathize with his neuroses, but he was just frightened. And—and he was very nice.

T: You became close with your father?

P: Well, as close as we could allow each other to be. We had this mutual love for the Brooklyn Dodgers, so he would take me to the games. Then we would always talk about it.

T: You and he?

P: Yes.

T: How old were you then?

P: Oh, I was 10—12—14. I felt sorry for him. I remember being at these Brooklyn Dodger games and I remember he couldn't demonstrate his feelings or let go of his feelings because he was a very avid fan. He couldn't . . . I remember my impulse when Jackie Robinson got a home run was to stand up and be excited by it, but I think I was intimidated more or less by my father being next to me. And he would get up very unenthusiastically and applaud. Do you know what I mean? Like he didn't have any excitement or enthusiasm.

T: Well how does that relate to you?

P: I think I started to behave like him.

T: Well, but in his relationship with you you say he didn't have excitement or show his feelings. How does that come into the relationship with you?

P: At that time?

T: Well in your life. In other words your father didn't show his feelings?

P: Yeah.

T: What I'm asking is how does that relate to you? You're saying that he didn't show his feelings in terms of you?

P: Yes. He didn't show his feelings . . .

T: Can you give me an example of that?

P: Well he never said to me that he loved me. I would do things for him to gain his affection. He would like these candy bars—fudge bars. So I would bring them to him, and he would always say "thank you," but that was as close as he could get. And it used to give me positive feelings or sometimes he would say "oh, you're a good boy" and that would make me feel good.

T: But you're feeling something right now.

P: Yes.

T: What are you experiencing?

P: A love for him or affection, but I guess a disappointment.

T: You're feeling something right now because there's a kind of catch in your voice and there's a tear in your eye.

P: I feel very emotional.

T: You feel it?

P: Yes.

T: Could you tell me what you're experiencing?

P: I feel close to my father and I feel also disappointed that it couldn't be more.

The interviewer then went on to examine the events leading to the father's death. What emerged was a description of the patient's father awakening in the middle of the night complaining of chest pain. The patient overheard his mother and father talking and sensed their distress. He went into their room and saw that his father looked pale and ashen, was holding his chest and seemed frightened. The patient immediately called for an ambulance. He accompanied his father to the hospital in the ambulance.

T: What was it like in the ambulance?

P: He was on a stretcher.

T: What did he look like?

P: Pale, sort of grey—sweating—not moving—lying on his back.

T: And what happened in the ambulance?

P: We talked—I remember he said the roads are unpaved or they have a lot of pot holes. Now I see it like he couldn't say or he wouldn't allow himself to say "I'm dying and I'm frightened." He would just like make this inappropriate small talk.

T: And what were you experiencing?

P: I was frightened that he was going to die. I was frightened and I didn't want him to die.

T: And as you're looking at this now you have this picture in your mind, what are you experiencing right now?

P: I would have liked to have held him and give him comfort.

T: To hold him how?

P: Embraced him. So we went to the hospital . . . (Patient attempts to move away from his tender feelings toward his father.)

T: Do you notice that you've moved away from your feelings? You would have liked to have embraced him?

P: Yes.

T: But you held back—you held on those feelings?

P: I held on them now.

T: You held on them—you kept away. Is that right?

P: Yes. I don't know if this is a rationalization, but he was not disposed to that kind of behavior and it would have made him anxious, I think.

T: So you felt that if you had done that, if you had embraced him—he would have what?

P: He would have been uncomfortable. He never embraced me. He did, but not with enthusiasm; or he couldn't allow himself to do that.

T: And then what happened? You got to the hospital?

P: Yes, he was rushed into this room, and a nurse was attending to him and then she left and I was just saying things like "do you want water?" or "how are you feeling?" And then he started like to fade, his breath became shallow and I ran out and got the nurse—I said you know take care of him, he's gonna die—he doesn't look good. So she came in and started administering to him. She got a doctor and then started doing things to him and then he died.

T: Did you have a chance to say good-bye?

P: No. I had a chance, but I didn't.

T: What are your feelings about that?

P: Sadness . . . I feel sad that . . . I feel sad that we weren't close. I think I feel sad because he didn't have any closeness in his life. He was sort of messed up. And it makes me feel sad. (Patient becomes tearful.)

T: So there is a tremendous yearning in you, this wish to have been closer, to have embraced him, to have said good-bye to him when he died?

P: Yes.

In this evaluation interview the therapist explored the patient's early relationship with his father. The patient's ambivalent and changing relationship with his father emerged. First, hostile, aggressive feelings were expressed, associated with the fantasy of wanting to kill his father in order to protect his mother. The therapist held the patient to this focus and did not allow him to digress. Details concerning these murderous feelings were elicited. Once the aggressive feelings toward his father were brought forth, the uncovering of positive feelings toward his father became possible. Again, details were elicited in a concrete manner through the use of a specific example, such as candy bars.

In both instances, the feelings clearly emerged: the angry, aggressive feelings, along with the loving, tender, and tearful ones. With the ambivalent feelings toward the father clearly expressed, the interviewer moved to an exploration of the father's actual death. Again, there is an emphasis on detailed exploration. The patient is asked to describe his father and what he looked like, both when he became sick and in the ambulance. This portraiting is extremely useful; it enables the patient to actively picture what he is describing so that the experience is relived. Patients will go through an intellectual experience that will have little therapeutic value unless their thoughts, memories, and affect are brought together.

Uncovering of repressed material is of great importance and becomes more feasible when minute details are focused upon. In a similar fashion, the funeral and burial should be closely examined.

Of particular significance is the therapist's emphasis on affect, which enables the patient to go through the mourning process. During the work of mourning, many specific memories concerning the lost object are explored, and the patient relives these experiences along with the appropriate emotions. It usually takes five to six sessions for the mourning process to be "completed."

Case Example "C"

A 37-year-old woman presented to the Center for Short-Term Dynamic Psychotherapy complaining of periodic panic attacks, multiple phobias, generalized anxiety, and a dissatisfaction with her marriage. Her panic attacks began more than 15 years earlier, and her phobias began a few years after that. She had been married for 14 years and had three children, ages 13, ten, and eight. She complained of her husband's lack of interest, yet felt she was undeserving of his love. Her mother died when she was six and her father remarried a year later. The patient had few memories about her mother. Her relationship with her father was mixed, alternating between care and longing for him, and hostile feelings associated with his lack of warmth and concern. There were primarily negative feelings toward her stepmother, which occasionally surfaced as criticisms or arguments.

During the initial interview, the interviewer attempted to focus on the mother's death. Despite a detailed inquiry, very little was learned about the mother, and the patient could not recall how she reacted or felt during the time of her mother's death. However, one important bit of information did emerge, indicating that the patient did not know where her mother was buried. The therapist underscored this, pointing out that she had kept this information from herself. The following are excerpts from the third, fifth and sixth psychotherapy sessions.

Third Session

In this session the focus was on the death of the patient's mother in the hospital.

P: I remember my father crying, but I can't—but I remember my father crying on a bus and I remember . . .

T: That would have been coming back from the hospital?

P: Probably—must have been coming back. I remember one visit with her that she had on a—she was in an oxygen tent. I remember that my father put a letter that she had gotten up on the tent so she could read it. Sometimes I think that, that fear, you know, is the same fear—maybe I was—in some way I was afraid—that seeing her closed in. Because a lot of my fears are of being closed in—of having something—of not being able to breathe.

T: So she was in an oxygen tent unable to breathe?

P: Right.

T: Having the type of difficulty that you now have.

P: Right—that's the memory that I have of her. But I don't really have any other memory.

T: So what did she—what did your mother look like?

The patient described her mother in some detail and the way she looked in the hospital, and became tearful. The therapist then asked about the funeral and burial, and this time the patient indicated that she was attempting to find out where her mother was buried. She obtained this information from a relative during the next two weeks. The fifth psychotherapy session centered on whether the patient would go to the cemetery and visit her mother's grave.

Fifth Session

P: I really don't want to go. I really don't want to go now.

T: You don't want to go.

P: I want to go somewhere and cry maybe.

T: Well, could we look at that? What are you feeling?

P: I'm just afraid. I don't . . .

T: Well it's important that we look at this because your relationship with your mother, your real mother is very, very important even though you have little in the way of memories about her. She was with you for those first six years and even the little we know about her indicates that she was a key person in your life and then she died. Our work together about your mother stimulated you to seek out where she was buried and now you feel like running away and again you put up a barrier. We were talking about that last time in relation to your father and Mark (her husband) and now you put up a barrier against your thoughts and feelings toward your mother.

P: No, I might go. I might go.

T: But do you see how you do that?

P: I just got used to the idea of going. I just got the location of the grave in the mail.

T: Still the hesitation.

P: Just, well I don't know quite what to do. I'm not sure . . .

T: Well look, one of the things that we know about you is that you suddenly develop fears, you get panicky and you run away. This doesn't seem to me to be so different from that.

P: My way out, I guess. I just run away . . . if I don't go I won't have to . . .

T: Well, do you want to get to the bottom of this?

P: Yes I do. But I'm . . .

T: But do you see then comes the barrier, the wall, the running away?

P: I can go. I can force myself to go.

T: But it's not the issue of whether you can—it's the issue what's going on inside you—you see?

P: Inside me I just have this fear of it a little bit.

T: Well, what is that all about?

P: I don't know what I'm going to find there. I don't know . . .

T: And what do you think you're going to find? What are you picturing?

P: All crumbled up (sobbing)—nobody ever took care of it— nobody ever . . .

T: You're going to find it neglected, a crumbled grave site?

P: I just feel bad that nobody ever went there all these years and never . . .

T: But you're saying nobody—who are you really talking about?

P: Nobody did.

T: But aren't you talking about yourself?

P: It's my father.

T: Well, but we're talking about you and you're the key person here.

P: Yeah, I guess. I just pretended like she didn't exist.

Sixth Session

P: I went to the cemetery, I think that was a strong thing, you know?

T: And what happened?

P: As they say—I survived.

T: You survived, but what else?

P: It was hard, it was hard to go.

T: You went by yourself?

P: Yeah. It was very hard to leave it. I had a lot of trouble going, but somehow I had a lot of trouble leaving. It was hard to find, for me to find the grave—it was just stupid. I don't know how to tell you this—it's just too much to tell you, but it was just—I don't know what to tell you but I went and it . . .

T: Well it's important that we take a look at it.

P: In some way I didn't feel like I was there. I had this just unreal feeling for part of it. I was watching myself but I wasn't feeling, you know, I wasn't there—I was there but I was . . .

T: You said you had trouble finding the grave site.

P: It was hot as hell that day. I went on Sunday when it was so hot.

T: And what was the trouble finding it?

P: I had it written down, so when I first went in I went to the office. There's an office there and the girl gave me a map and she circled the number and showed me where it was. It's like a big block—like a city block. And then my aunt had written a certain gate and row number. So, when I got to the block I just thought I'd be able to walk and find it, you know. So I just walked, but I couldn't find it that way. And then I looked for this gate—they have different archways there. Then I saw writing which I couldn't read and I just got all nervous, I just—I—somehow I didn't see it. I walked all around—I sort of looked at the gates and I just couldn't see the one I was looking for. I had to go all the way back to the office again. Then I went back and the girl said it's written on the gate—how could I not see it? I said well please draw it for me, just where it is—I couldn't find it. So she drew it and that time when I went back I found it.

T: It was on the gate—the number?

P: It was on the gate. I just didn't see it. But the gates have a lot of parts—they have the part that opens and the archway. There's a lot of writing on it.

T: Well, we know that there's a part of you that was reluctant to go in the first place. Was this still part of it?

P: No, no I don't think so. I don't think—I don't know. Anyway I . . .

T: But you persisted?

P: I did. I went back and I just thought I would know it somehow. When I first went . . .

T: What happened?

P: Well, I caught sight of it and something electrical almost when I saw her name there.

T: Her name is?

P: Emily. Emily. And I went over to it and it was very crowded—there wasn't very much room, but it is there. And it had something very nice written on it. It said 'a little bit of sunshine, of joy lies here' (sobbing). And it wasn't on any other grave. I looked at a lot of graves. Before I even got there I cried a lot because of just being in the cemetery—I guess I just kept getting lost and some of the children's graves (waves of sobbing). Just walking, row and row and row it just seemed so endless. There was nobody else there—I saw two other people in that whole place—it was like a desert—and anyway—and so I saw her birthday which is the—she's the same sign as I am, May 10th. A few things I didn't know—the exact day when she had died, which I had known. And some writing on it and I just—I said the prayer. There's this little book you can get in the office and I said the prayer. Then I put some stones on the grave.

T: So you said a prayer and put stones on the grave.

P: First I put one—there was a stone on there. I put one and I came back and found another one I liked better. I couldn't leave—it was very hard to leave it. And then after I was leaving I found a real pretty, little white one and I went back and put that on too—it looked like more people were there.

T: Why did you want it to look like more people were there?

P: I didn't really—I think I just . . .

T: Because when we talked about it last time you said that you felt guilty that the grave might be neglected and that you had neglected to visit it.

P: I know. I sort of—I don't know.

T: Did you still have that feeling when you were there?

P: I did. I . . .

T: Did it looked neglected?

P: It didn't look too bad. It had some ivy planted in a planter.

T: So when you got there it didn't look neglected?

P: No. It didn't look as old as I thought. Before I had been going up to the real old, dark stone ones because I figured it was so far back, but it wasn't old looking. When I first saw it I just felt a shock—I don't know. I knew I was going to it—it was just a funny feeling for a minute, you know. I wasn't near it—I was in the middle path and I just saw it over there—I knew it was the fifth one. When I just saw her name there.

T: And the prayer you said was what?

P: The Mourner's Prayer and a prayer you're supposed to say for your mother.

T: And what were you thinking while you were there?

P: I was talking to her really.

T: Saying what?

P: Just—I don't remember the words—I just felt very sad—I told her one stone was for my father 'cause he really thinks about her a lot, even if he doesn't seem to. I don't know—I was trying to say good-bye because that's what I felt I really came for (sobbing).

T: And?

P: I don't know—I don't know. It's still very mixed up, my feelings about it.

T: Well what are the feelings?

P: I'm glad it's over—I don't think I'll go back again, at least for awhile.

T: What are the mixed feelings?

P: I don't know who I'm saying good-bye to and what I went to accomplish really. It wasn't really that clear in my mind—I just went to see what I would feel and whatever would come.

T: Well clearly you felt a lot?

P: The same old sadness.

T: The sadness, the loss? But the feeling that her grave was neglected is gone?

P: Yeah. I'm sorry she was so crowded in. I was thinking that I would like to be buried there, but there's no room.

T: What made you think that you'd like to be buried there?

P: I have to be buried somewhere.

T: You thought of it then or just now?

P: When I got there. I was sad it was so crowded. I knelt down but you really didn't have enough room. By the time I got up I could hardly stand—my feet were just asleep you know, from being in one position so long.

T: So there's no room for you there?

P: No. Not next to her. No. It's so ridiculous—I kissed the stone (sobbing) thinking that there was somebody there—there's nobody there. I think I still think somebody's there.

It is significant that this patient was able to experience the mourning process 31 years after the death of her mother. The patient had not been able to mourn her mother's death at age six or at any other time. She remembered little about her mother or her mother's death. The therapeutic task of uncovering this material led to the question of where her mother was buried. The patient pursued this question and finally visited the grave. This was made possible by the therapist consistently confronting the resistances and focusing on the mother's death.

The patient found the burial site, but was ambivalent about going to the cemetery. The therapist interpreted her reluctance to go to the cemetery as erecting a barrier against her mother. What emerged were the patient's feelings of guilt about not visiting and not caring for the grave. This was expressed through the metaphor of a crumbled grave site, indicating her guilt and underlying anger toward her mother for leaving and neglecting her.

Her visit to the cemetery brings the mourning process into high gear. Sobbing occurs in waves as a great many details about her mother and the grave emerge. The patient sees her mother's name, the inscription, says a prayer for the dead, and one for her mother. She is reluctant to leave and ends by kissing the tombstone (mother). During the next several sessions, the mourning for her mother is worked through, allowing the therapy to turn to other issues.

SUMMARY

This chapter reviews some of the psychoanalytic thinking about mourning. The stages of normal mourning are presented and differentiated from pathological mourning.

It is critical that pathological mourning be recognized during the evaluation interview so that it can be explored early in psychotherapy. If this is not done, the pathological mourning becomes a barrier to therapeutic progress in other areas of the patient's life.

The techniques used in short-term dynamic psychotherapy are ideally suited to uncover and work through pathological mourning. The emphasis is on the examination of the lost object, including a concrete and detailed exploration of the death, funeral, and burial. Portraiting or painting these pictures helps the patient to relive the experience. It is important that the experience be accompanied by affect, so that the mourning process can occur. Both positive and negative feelings for the lost object must be uncovered and brought into the mourning process and worked through before turning to other issues.

References

1. Murphy W: The Tactics of Psychotherapy. The Application of Psychoanalytic Therapy to Psychotherapy. New York, International Universities Press, 1965

2. Davanloo H: The technique of crisis evaluation and intervention, in Short-Term Dynamic Psychotherapy. Edited by Davanloo H. New York, Jason Aronson, 1980

3. Freud S: Mourning and melancholia (1917), in Complete Psychological Works, Standard Edition, vol. 14. Translated and edited by Strachey J. London, Hogarth Press, 1961

4. Abraham K: A short study of the development of the libido, viewed in the light of mental disorders, in Selected Papers on Psychoanalysis. London, Hogarth Press, 1924

5. Lindemann E: Symptomatology and management of acute grief. Psychiatry 47:14-25, 1944

6. Bowlby J: Pathological mourning and childhood mourning. J Am Psychoanal Assoc 11:500-549, 1963

7. Winston A, Goldin V: Pathological mourning and short-term dynamic psychotherapy. American Psychiatric Association 137th Annual Meeting, Syllabus and Scientific Proceedings. Los Angeles, May 1984

8. Loewald H: Internalization, separation, mourning and the superego. Psychoanal Q 31:483-504, 1962

9. Mahler M, Pine F, Bergman A: The Psychological Birth of the Human Infant. New York, Basic Books, 1975

10. Horowitz M, Wilner N, Marmar C, et al: Pathological grief and the activation of latent self-images. Am J Psychiatry 137:1157-1162, 1980

11. Brown J, Stoudemire A: Normal and pathological grief. JAMA 250:379-382, 1983

12. Joffe W, Sandler J: Notes on pain, depression and individuation. Psychoanal Study Child 20:394-424, 1965

13. Gorkin M: Narcissistic personality disorder and pathological mourning. Contemporary Psychoanalysis 20:400-420, 1984

14. Klein M: On the theory of anxiety and guilt, in Developments in Psychoanalysis. Edited by Rivere J. London, Hogarth Press, 1952

15. Deutsch H: Absence of Grief. Psychoanal Q 6:12-22, 1937

16. Ferenczi S: The problem of acceptance of unpleasant ideas: advances in the knowledge of the sense of reality, in Further Contributions to the Theory and Technique of Psychoanalysis. New York, Basic Books, 1960

17. Kohut H: The Analysis of the Self. New York, International Universities Press, 1971

18. Davanloo H: A method of short-term dynamic psychotherapy, in Short-Term Dynamic Psychotherapy. Edited by Davanloo H. New York, Jason Aronson, 1980

19. Davanloo H: Response to interpretation, in Short-Term Dynamic Psychotherapy. Edited by Davanloo H. New York, Jason Aronson, 1980

3

Brief Adaptation-Oriented Psychotherapy

Jerome Pollack, M.D.
Althea Horner, Ph.D.

3

Brief Adaptation-Oriented Psychotherapy

Brief adaptation-oriented psychotherapy is a method of short-term therapy that was devised in a research project at Beth Israel Medical Center. It was designed to be used as a comparison to short-term dynamic psychotherapy based on the work of Davanloo (1). The full research project is an attempt to delineate the important specific events in psychotherapy that lead to the therapeutic efficacy of the treatment. This is in contrast to the work of Frank (2) and Strupp (3), which emphasizes the role of nonspecific factors in psychotherapy.

Both brief adaptation-oriented psychotherapy and short-term dynamic psychotherapy investigate whether short-term approaches can, in general, be therapeutic. These treatment approaches examine ways in which resistances can be handled to allow the therapeutic alliance to be more effective, and seek out ways to interpret transference resistances. Both approaches attempt to avoid a transference neurosis or enmeshment, which leads to greater dependence on the therapist, making a short-term approach impossible. In addition, brief adaptation-oriented psychotherapy and short-term dynamic psychotherapy search for alternative ways to determine the major focus of the treatment. These forms of therapy also examine the relative importance of cognitive versus affective components in the interventions made by the therapists. Brief adaptation-oriented psychotherapy is primarily a cognitive therapy, while short-term dynamic psychotherapy involves more work done by the therapist in order to evoke the patient's affect during the therapy. It should be noted that both treatments work with cognitive and affective factors; the difference between them is the relative emphasis placed on each.

THE DEVELOPMENT OF BRIEF ADAPTATION-ORIENTED PSYCHOTHERAPY

Brief adaptation-oriented psychotherapy was developed out of the long-standing tradition of psychoanalysis, psychoanalytic psychotherapy, and ego psychology. It has also incorporated such methods of short-term psychotherapy as those developed by Ferenczi (4), Alexander and French (5), Murphy (6), Malan (7), and Sifneos (9). Our goal was to take long-term psychoanalytic psychotherapy and find ways to make it less open-ended and thereby briefer, without sacrificing its essence or its therapeutic efficacy.

The major principles of brief adaptation-oriented psychotherapy rely heavily on the concepts of the dynamic unconscious, early conflict as an important source of character formation, the relationship of character to adaptation (and maladaptive behavior), the importance of the transference in psychotherapy, and the use of interpretation to give the patient insight into his or her adaptation and thus allow change to occur.

Importance of the Time Limit

In brief adaptation-oriented psychotherapy, as in short-term dynamic psychotherapy, patients are seen for a maximum of 40 sessions, once a week. This allows the treatment to continue, providing time for change to occur while the patient is still in the active therapeutic process. This also allows time for working through, so that the patient can make the beginnings of different adaptations while in therapy, and the change can be monitored effectively. In formulating brief adaptation-oriented psychotherapy, we wanted to stay away from the shorter approaches, such as

Mann's (8), because we feel that therapies of 12 sessions or less tend to fix the therapeutic focus on issues of separation and loss. While issues of separation and loss are ubiquitous, they are neither the only issues nor the issues we want to work with exclusively. We do not want to be limited in that direction; longer therapy has the advantage of opening up issues that can be used as the primary focus.

No minimum number of sessions was set when we first implemented brief adaptation-oriented psychotherapy. In our experience, however, the full 40 sessions are necessary. There are a number of reasons for this. We were devising a new system of therapy, and training therapists in the use of a new, unfamiliar, technique. Therefore, interventions usually came later than they might have if the therapists were more familiar with the technique. There were also problems with the selection of patients, which is a crucial factor in short-term therapy, as indicated in the work of Davanloo (1), Malan (7), and Sifneos (9). Probably the most important factor in determining the length of the therapy, however, was the reluctance of therapists to be as active as is necessary in a brief approach; and, related to this, the fact that therapists trained in long-term therapy are often reluctant to look upon short-term approaches with real expectations for success. This is true even if they are training in the new technique. Frank (2) demonstrates that one essential factor in the success of psychotherapy is the belief of the therapist in the system of therapy. Though this is difficult to measure, it is a factor to be considered. A more accurate appraisal would be possible after a therapist has treated a number of cases.

It is most important that both the patient and the therapist know that there is a limit to the number of sessions and that the limit will be adhered to. This is very effective in limiting the number of missed sessions, and in having the patient and the therapist spend less time on issues outside the major focus. It induces much greater activity within the session and makes both the patient and the therapist less tolerant of tangential issues.

The spectre of a finite number of sessions is always present. A useful intervention on the part of the therapist is often, "If you do not stick to our mutually agreed-upon focus, the number of sessions will add up and we will be left at the end of treatment not having fully explored the problem you came here for." It is inevitable in the therapy that at some time past the midpoint the patient displays anger at being limited in the number of sessions, and questions whether any exceptions can be made. There is no doubt that both the therapist and the patient are always aware of the limited number of sessions, and that this is a spur to a more active therapy. If the patient wants to continue therapy, he or she is asked to wait for six months, if at all possible, because we have found that therapeutic change continues to take place after formal therapy is over. This has also been reported by such researchers in the field as Davanloo (1) and Sifneos (9). A process is started in the therapy that can continue even after the therapy is over; the need for further therapy may, therefore, be obviated.

THE GOAL OF BRIEF ADAPTATION-ORIENTED PSYCHOTHERAPY

Any short-term psychotherapy must have some attainable therapeutic goal. It cannot be a general goal, such as being able to love or work more effectively, but must be specific and realistically attainable within a fixed period of time. In brief adaptation-oriented psychotherapy, the therapeutic goal is to change the major maladaptive pattern of the patient. Since the orientation is psychoanalytic and ego psychological, the premise is that in order to accomplish therapeutic change with some lasting effect, the therapist must help the patient to do something that will focus on his or her usual style of living; that is, on the patient's mode of adaptation. The therapist cannot change a patient's environment or world. But the therapist can work with the patient to help change the way in which the patient responds to the environment; that is, to alter the patient's defensive organization and character. It would be arrogant to claim that in a period of 40 sessions, brief adaptation-oriented psychotherapy can significantly alter the total character structure of a patient. Our psychoanalytic colleagues spend years with their analysands and wonder whether they can accomplish this goal. However, the question we are examining is whether we can take one pattern of the patient's responses to the internal and external world, examine it in microscopic fashion, and have the patient alter that pattern so that behavior becomes more adaptive, allowing life to become more effective.

Adaptation

Broadly speaking, adaptation is the integration of beliefs, wishes, needs, and impulses with the demands of the external world and the demands of the superego. The core issue of adaptation is internal and external reality. A knowledge of reality and acting in accordance with it leads to the achievement of a maximum amount of gratification with a minimum amount of pain (Hartmann 10). The failure of this integration by the ego may result in maladaptive patterns of behavior, which, in some cases, leads to the formation of personality disorders.

Personality traits, in themselves, are not considered mental disorders. They may include such factors as innate temperament or cognitive style. *DSM-III* (11) defines personality traits as "enduring patterns of perceiving, relating to, and thinking about the environment and oneself . . . " However, these traits may, and often do, become rigid in an attempt at adaptation. When they become inflexible and maladaptive they are referred to as personality disorders. When traits serve adaptation, all is fine; but when they add to maladaptive patterns that do not serve present reality and adaptation, they must be loosened, examined microscopically, and altered to serve the present reality. In brief adaptation-oriented psychotherapy, one does not challenge an obsessive or hysteric style per se; one challenges that style as it relates to the maladaptive pattern. Our goal is to alter the personality trait so that it becomes less rigid, and more adaptive than maladaptive.

Adaptation takes place under the aegis of the ego. Brief adaptation-oriented psychotherapy is an ego psychological approach, exploring ways in which the ego deals with wishes, beliefs, needs, and impulses, both adaptively (that is, consistent with the present reality) and maladaptively (not consistent with the present reality).

The therapist must, therefore, examine all the factors that enter into the maladaptive pattern: the thoughts, perceptions, feelings, beliefs, or wishes, to see whether they contain areas of conflict and reality distortion. We know enough about character and personality to understand that they are derived from previous conflicts during development (11). While the elements of the pattern may have served adaptation when they were developed, they do not serve present reality and have become rigid, thus no longer serving adaptation. A woman who, as a girl, accommodated totally to her parents' wishes as an adaptational maneuver does not serve the present reality when she accommodates to all of her boss's wishes now that she is an adult. While her accommodating behavior might have served adaptation at one point in her life, the anger that it occasions in the present, and the need to defend against this anger, no longer serves adaptation; it is now a maladaptive pattern that must be explored. The pattern must be taken out of its rigid position and altered to conform to the present reality, both internal and external. We can see the ways in which the patient reacts to the present reality on the basis of past maladaptive patterns.

Use of Brief Adaptation-Oriented Psychotherapy to Change Maladaptive Patterns

Brief adaptation-oriented psychotherapy focuses on these maladaptive patterns that are rigid, enduring patterns of perceiving, relating to, and thinking about the environment and the self, as well as the behaviors based on these patterns. Examples of major maladaptive patterns are:

1. The wish to be "special," and the belief that one has to accommodate to the other in order to be special. This may lead to a loss of assertiveness and the undermining of the possibility for success.
2. The wish to succeed, which may generate the fear of competitiveness and fear of being envied by others. This can lead

to the maladaptive behaviors of passivity, inaction, and dependency.

3. The wish to be taken care of, which leads to feelings of shame and loss of self-esteem. The maladaptive defense can be playing caretaker to everyone else, leading to resentment that one is not being taken care of in return.

4. The fear that one's aggression or self-assertion will lead to the loss of wished-for love. This may lead to withdrawal from conflict as soon as it appears and to overly compliant behavior.

Our approach is to expose the specific major maladaptive pattern in order to elucidate the ways in which it operates in the present, especially within the patient's important relationships. One of the principal therapeutic tools involves questioning the patient so that the maladaptive pattern can be dissected into its elements, which are:

1. The wish;
2. The beliefs associated with the wish;
3. The consequences of the wish;
4. Conflicts between wishes;
5. The defensive posture brought on by the conflicts.

These make up the structure of the pattern. It is the task of the patient and therapist to bring to light the structure of the maladaptive pattern in all of its manifestations, past and present, with the therapist leading the way. The method is constant confrontation of the patient, asking him or her to look further into the various elements and not be satisfied by general statements that tend to obfuscate the true nature of the wishes and beliefs. The resistance comes to the fore in various ways at this point, and the therapeutic relationship must stand its severest test. Often there are wishes on the part of the patient to leave therapy, to evade issues, to talk about truisms that have no specific meaning to the patient, and to use the defensive posture that is a part of the maladaptive pattern. If the patient has been well selected and is motivated to be in treatment, the patient will not drop out and will respond to the therapist's examination of the pathology in all of its elements. The resistance at this point can be directly dealt with as part of the transference; that is, the attempts of the patient to see the therapist as an important figure from the past (usually the parent), and a direct interpretation of this, can be made.

It is essential that the therapist bring himself or herself into the treatment early, by relating some of the patient's material to the person of the therapist. This is done by asking the patient as he or she is discussing a part of the pattern: "How does that work in here?" This is a way of conveying to the patient, from the beginning, that the therapist will be looking at all manifestations of the patient's relationships, including the therapeutic relationship. The goal is to show the patient that the maladaptive pattern is global, that it stands in the way of achieving life goals, and that it hinders the imparting of information to the therapist, thus preventing treatment goals from being reached.

By subjecting specific ways of perceiving, relating to, and thinking about the environment and the self to intense scrutiny, and thus to reality testing, the patient may be brought more closely in line with the present reality, rendering the patient's pattern more adaptive. With insight into the role of these patterns in the patient's overall psychological economy, he or she is given the opportunity to give up the maladaptive patterns of thinking, feeling, perceiving, and behaving and, instead, to substitute a more adaptive, reality-oriented mode of functioning to a degree sufficient to bring about significant change.

Brief adaptation-oriented psychotherapy's working hypothesis is that if the distortions of the adaptive process are made accessible to the ego's reality testing (a function that is intact in our patient population) the ego will be able to formulate a new, reality-oriented adaptation. Examination of the specific distortions of the patient's adaptive attempts will enable the patient to understand the ways in which what were once adaptive processes may now be maladaptive. Once this understanding is achieved, the patient can work on changing these patterns so that they may, once again, become adaptive in the patient's current reality. However, what must be kept in mind is that brief adaptation-oriented psychotherapy is psychodynamically based psychotherapy, with more of an allegiance to the ego psychological, psychoanalytic approach (Hartmann 10), as opposed to cognitive therapy (13), which is based on behavior modification. It is brief adaptation-oriented psychotherapy's goal to show the patient the distortions of the adaptation process in relationships, to show the patient that this is based on adaptations developed during the formative years, and that this continued way of responding to the environment gets in the way of achieving goals, especially in regard to important current relationships.

SELECTING PATIENTS FOR BRIEF ADAPTATION-ORIENTED PSYCHOTHERAPY

The selection of patients is an important factor in any short-term therapy (1, 9, 14). One must select patients who will benefit from the therapy, and who are able to work in an intensive treatment utilizing an active dissection of thought and behavior. The project for which brief adaptation-oriented psychotherapy was developed stipulates that the patient population be among the following diagnostic categories, using *DSM-III* (11) as the classification: Dependent Personality Disorder (301.60); Histrionic Personality Disorder (301.50); Compulsive Personality Disorder (301.40); Passive-Aggressive Personality Disorder (301.84); Avoidant Personality Disorder (301.82); and Atypical, Mixed or other Personality Disorder (301.89). Rarely does one see a pure culture of a personality disorder; therefore, the Mixed category was included. Some personality disorders are specifically ruled out, such as the Borderline, Narcissistic and Antisocial classifications. These disorders are not amenable to a short-term approach at the present time. This is not to say that these disorders may not be treated using a short-term approach: if a different goal of treatment were defined, there could be a therapeutic benefit. However, at our stage of expertise with brief adaptation-oriented psychotherapy, trying to treat these disorders could cloud the issue and add too many parameters. Other contraindications are used in an attempt to gather a clinical population with which our therapists (all of whom are new to the technique) can be comfortable using a short-term approach. These contraindications are:

1. Suicide potential (as contrasted with suicidal thoughts). We excluded all patients who exhibited suicidal behavior;
2. Severe acting out—legal problems, sociopathic behavior;
3. Addictive problems—excessive use of drugs or alcohol, or eating disorders (anorexia or bulimia);
4. Total absence of anxiety (alexythymia);
5. Psychosis, or any history of psychotic episodes;
6. Absence of an altruistic relationship;
7. Inability to use the cognitive mode—for example, retardation, excessive concreteness;
8. Lack of psychological mindedness—inability to see connections of one piece of behavior to another, especially casual connections;
9. Use of a major tranquilizer or antidepressant that the patient is unable to give up;
10. Paranoid tendencies.

The Evaluation Interview

Patients are chosen with whom our therapists can work comfortably. This necessitates a full evaluation of the patient, consisting of at least one interview that is a minimum of two hours long, before a patient can be accepted for treatment. A long interview tends to be quite stressful for the patient; observing the patient under this type of stress gives us some understanding of the patient's ego, and gives us an indication as to whether the patient can benefit from an active approach without serious regression and/or acting out. Most patients have two evaluation interviews, each lasting two hours.

The interviewer is expected to get a complete psychiatric history and to assay the ego of the patient. Once all contraindications are ruled out, the interviewer focuses on the major maladaptive pattern and confronts the patient with it. At this point in the interview, the therapist cannot expect total agreement on the part of the patient. This would be expected only in an overly compliant patient. Instead, it is hoped that the patient will respond to the confrontation and provide more information. The patient often demonstrates the maladaptive pattern in another area, or understands the ways in which the pattern has been maladaptive. If the patient disagrees with the pattern that the interviewer presents, the response itself could elucidate other aspects of maladaptive behavior. In our experience, the pattern presented at the beginning of therapy is often not the final pattern elucidated during treatment. There are changes as more data is presented in the ongoing process of treatment.

The therapist's task in the beginning of therapy is to make sure that the patient is able to work with the technique, is able to form a therapeutic alliance with the therapist, and is able to progress from there. It is important that the patient immediately see the therapy as a vigorous, investigative approach to his or her verbalizations, and can tolerate the pursuit of what lies beyond the obvious and the superficial. The ideal patient will not only tolerate this, but will join in the process. The training of the patient to do this type of work must start in the evaluation session. It is not just a fact gathering session; it is the beginning of the therapy. From that point on, neither the patient nor the therapist can take a passive stance. The patient must be confronted from the start. General statements should not pass; the therapist must find out specifics. The therapist should not be reluctant to bring himself or herself into the material. Any allusion to the therapist should be confronted, and the patient should be asked to enlarge upon it. If the beginning therapist is reluctant to do this, the therapeutic relationship will be left out of the maladaptive pattern.

It is hoped that the therapist, by the end of the evaluation, will have a good idea of the major maladaptive pattern, of the defensive organization, of possible resistances, and of the quality of the therapeutic alliance. The therapist presents the patient with the major maladaptive pattern and proposes that they start to work, elucidating the way this pattern operates, what its components are, where it all started, and how it affects the patient's life. It is also in the evaluation interview that the patient is apprised of the rules (which are similar to the rules of any psychoanalytic psychotherapy) and told that there will be a maximum of 40 sessions.

EXAMINATION OF THE THERAPEUTIC RELATIONSHIP

The examination of the therapeutic relationship and its relation to the major maladaptive pattern is the cornerstone of brief adaptation-oriented psychotherapy. The therapeutic relationship is an important relationship, it is in the here and now, and it is subject to all of the distortions that the patient uses in other relationships. The exclusion of the therapeutic relationship would weaken any therapy that is examining the interpersonal relationships in the life of the patient. The object is to understand the pattern of the patient, to examine the ramifications of this pattern throughout the life of the patient (including its origins), to see the ways in which this pattern manifests itself in other areas of the patient's life (both present and past), and to see how this pattern is manifested in the relationship between the patient and therapist.

The therapist's consistent failure to question the patient's hints relating to the therapeutic relationship conveys a message to the patient to ignore this relationship. All this will serve to give the patient some intellectualized, cognitive insight, but this is not what the treatment is intended to be. Any allusion to the therapist must be explored by the patient, and the therapist must actively encourage the patient to do this at any point in the treatment, including the initial evaluation.

A difficult type of patient is one who accommodates to the therapist, agrees to every intervention made, and yet does not alter behavior. It appears as if the patient has a positive transference, which, however, turns out to be antitherapeutic. Gill (15) has written about this phenomenon. Early intervention concerning the nature of the therapeutic relationship is mandatory in this type of patient, or there will be no real change in the patient. Forty sessions will pass, and the patient will leave as he or she came, still accommodating in every relationship. The most effective way to combat this is direct exposure within the treatment to the nature of the therapeutic relationship—how the patient relates to the therapist using the old ways—which have been maladaptive in the past, and are maladaptive in the treatment. All three aspects of this are crucial in brief adaptation-oriented psychotherapy, and any therapeutic effect depends on pursuit of these factors. Our task is to constantly pursue the elements of the pattern, asking patients to explore all facets of the maladaptive pattern and to combat resistance as it appears. Then, when the pattern is presented and when its operation in the therapeutic relationship is clear, the therapist must interpret this to the patient a la Strachey (16), with the psychodynamics of the past, the present, and the transference.

PUTTING THE TREATMENT INTO PRACTICE

Psychoanalytic psychotherapy is often long-term and open-ended because of the regression that occurs in the patient during this type of treatment. One of the factors to be avoided in brief psychotherapies is the dependent relationship that develops in the transference. The purpose in classical psychoanalytic treatment is to allow a transference neurosis to develop that is the inheritor of the infantile neurosis (along with other factors in the early life of the patient) and to intensively analyze this on a long-term basis in order to terminate therapy. While this can be of immense value, psychoanalysis cannot be used in treating all of the patients who need treatment. Not everyone can enter into analysis, and, in fact, there are not enough analysts to go around. Both brief adaptation-oriented psychotherapy and short-term dynamic psychotherapy are designed to see whether we can achieve therapeutic results—real changes that are long lasting—using shorter approaches, and can put these approaches into operation using a psychoanalytic model.

Certainly an important part of the answer is to avoid the regression of the transference neurosis (an important factor in the structure of psychoanalysis) by not allowing it to develop. This can be done by interpreting any material that may relate to the transference early in the treatment. If a patient makes an allusion to a past therapy, it must be explored as it compares to the present therapy. If the material that the patient presents relates to relationships with past figures, especially parents, the therapist must see how this relates to the treatment relationship and explore this with the patient. The therapist must constantly be on guard, looking for regressive phenomena such as dependence and passivity, and must explore this to see how it is manifested in the present and in the therapy. Continual exploration of these factors is often effective in the prevention of regression, prevents the formation of a transference neurosis, and makes possible a shorter approach that may still result in long-term therapeutic gains.

The Sessions

All the evaluation and therapy sessions were videotaped, and there was one-to-one supervision of all sessions by the authors. In addition, there were weekly conferences where all evaluations were screened and the therapists would come to some agreement as to the suitability of the patient for brief adaptation-oriented psychotherapy, the major maladaptive pattern, and the possible difficulties of the treatment. An attempt was made to have the therapists see therapy sessions of other therapists, so that a critique of the treatment could be done. This was invaluable in putting the treatment into operation and forming a cohesive group of therapists, all trying to solve problems found with the treatment. The supervisors had to constantly work on a number of factors, even with rather experienced therapists. These included getting the therapists to maintain the focus, relating the productions to the major maladaptive pattern, and having the therapists bring up the transference early in the treatment, where applicable.

Case Example One

The patient was a 36-year-old married woman, mother of two children, who came to treatment because of an inability to have a satisfactory sexual relationship with her husband. This had been present throughout the marriage. The patient was an attorney and complained that she was always working harder than her associates and never reaping the benefits of her work.

The major maladaptive pattern that was determined early in the treatment was her need to accommodate to all the demands of the important people in her life. She did this in response to demands made by her husband, her bosses, her siblings, and her children, even though she knew that accommodating all their demands might not serve either her needs or theirs. The patient indulged all the people in her life, but this led to a great deal of anger that she could never express. She would retire after confrontations and cry out her feelings in private. In public she would maintain a girlish, somewhat stoical image.

The pattern, that of smiling accommodation to all the demands of others, was very apparent in the transference. She would report all her actions to the therapist, all in the same girlish manner. The therapist chose to confront her concerning what lay underneath her accommodations to everyone. He quickly learned that she had had a lover for about three months. They had a satisfactory sexual relationship, but she accommodated totally to his wishes. The situation was that she had a husband to whom she felt close personally, but not sexually; and a lover to whom she felt close sexually, but with whom she felt she could never have a long-term relationship in any but a sexual way.

She characterized herself as having a "whore-madonna" split. She felt sexually stimulated by one man and was a madonna to another (her husband). This was worked back to a long-term boyfriend she had before marriage who was very satisfying to her sexually. She did not marry him, since he was a "ladies' man," and she felt he would never be faithful. It soon emerged that this related to her father, an alcoholic who died when she was 12 and who was closer to her older sisters than he was to her. Their closeness was a source of great disappointment to the patient. She was able to trace back to this situation her great feelings of vulnerability and disappointment in men. She would never be able to give herself totally to a man, and would always hold something in reserve, as she had done all her life. This was brought into the therapeutic relationship by the therapist pointing out, quite early in the therapy, that the patient could not show her feelings to him, and, in fact, that the patient related to the therapist in an accommodating, girlish way and not as a mature woman. She related to the therapist in the same way as she related to her husband, lover, boss, and father. This was followed by some acting out on the part of the patient. She missed a couple of sessions, which the therapist saw as confirming his interpretation. It was later confirmed when, at the end of therapy, the patient pointed out that she had thought the therapist, like her father, was an alcoholic, and she felt she could not trust the therapist because of that.

The patient was able to see her pattern in operation in all the important relationships in the present, the past, and in the transference. As a result of this she was able to see the relationship with her lover as being a partial one (he also looked like her father) and was able to try to make her marriage work, if at all possible. The patient was able to terminate after 40 sessions.

Case Example Two

The patient was a 50-year-old woman who came to treatment because of an inability to make a long-term commitment either in work or in relationships with men. She had worked most of her adult life in a variety of jobs in various fields, never staying in any one job for any length of time, and never feeling satisfied with any of them. She had a number of relationships with men, including two marriages, but again none were satisfactory for any length of time. Despite these difficulties she managed to maintain herself in reasonably comfortable circumstances, had friends of long duration, and had the capacity to enjoy a variety of experiences. The patient had multiple therapies in a variety of modalities for a large part of her adult life, for problems similar to those that brought her to treatment this time.

The major maladaptive pattern was conceived to be the patient's unwillingness to commit herself to anything that mattered to her; that is, jobs and men. This was connected to her father's leaving her. The patient's father and mother had a stormy marriage marked by many separations. The final one took place when she was pre-adolescent. The father was an alcoholic to whom the patient was very close and who she described as being "a lot of fun." He had, however, deserted her, and subsequently died. Her maladaptive behavior centered around not wanting anything, and not committing herself to anything, so that she would not be disappointed.

At the same time there was the underlying fantasy that her father was not dead (she did not go to the funeral and in fact did not know where he was buried), and that he would return someday and make everything all right again. Hence, there was no urgency to solve her problems and no need to make a long-term commitment to anything.

At the start of therapy the patient began a new job, and the early sessions dealt mainly with the patient's many complaints about the job and her wish to quit. In the sixth session she realized that she couldn't trust her boss, which led to memories of being unable to trust either her mother or father. Her pattern of running away from situations where she could be hurt, as she had been by her father, was pointed out to her in relation to the job, which, though not ideal, seemed to have things in its favor. In the next session, she reported that she had left the job. Because the therapist had taken the position of encouraging her to see whether the job could work out, she had quit the job in order to devalue the role of the therapist and was, in fact, distancing herself from him. She quit the job rather than see all of its ramifications.

The main work of the next sessions dealt with the interpretation of her defense of distancing herself in her personal life and in the transference. In session 11, the patient reported feeling hopeless. She expected more from therapy. This was related to her fantasy concerning the return of her father to make everything better, and the disappointment in the therapist as a substitute. The patient remained in treatment, and more and more material about her childhood relationship with her parents was produced. Her ambivalence toward both her mother and father came to the fore. Again, this was related to her need to distance herself in order to avoid conflict and disappointment in her life and in the transference.

A great deal of anger, as well as her fear of this anger, came through in the 30th to 35th sessions. Her fear of anger was related to death wishes toward the mother, and the fear of losing her as she had lost her father in reality. She then reported that she had been working at a job that was quite satisfactory to her and that seemed to be a good career opportunity. Until the end of therapy she continued to have difficulty in expressing feelings of anger toward the therapist, but was able to express angry feelings toward others. She was able to talk about termination with sad feelings about missing the therapist.

The last sessions dealt with her relationships with men, which were still tenuous. The original fantasy of waiting for the father reemerged in the idea that if she couldn't have a perfect man, she'd rather have none. While the patient was able to show real sadness about terminating therapy and stated she would miss the therapist, she maintained some distance throughout the closing sessions.

SUMMARY

Brief adaptation-oriented psychotherapy is a short-term therapy based on psychoanalytic and ego psychological models that has been derived from other methods of short-term psychotherapy.

Patients are seen for a maximum of forty (40) sessions once a week. The major focus of the therapy is the primary maladaptive pattern. The object is to microscopically dissect the pattern into its components, thus affording the patient insight into the maladaptation. The pattern is looked at from the point of view of its development, its operation in the major relationships of the patient, and its operation in the therapeutic relationship. Brief adaptation-oriented psychotherapy has been applied until now to personality disorders, and the patients have been carefully selected. The application of this method to other pathological conditions remains to be determined.

There is an acknowledged need in dynamic psychiatry to shorten the duration of psychotherapy. There are enormous pressures on our discipline brought to bear by governmental funding agencies, insurance companies, and the general public. The question is, how can we make a psychoanalytically based psychotherapy better and more accessible to both the public and the professional community? Can we train therapists well versed in psychoanalytic psychotherapy in another, complementary, yet rigorous technique, so that they can be therapeutic in a shorter period of time? Can we treat more patients and still achieve effective results? These are the questions we are seeking to answer.

References

1. Davanloo H: Basic Principles and Techniques in Short-Term Dynamic Psychotherapy. New York, Spectrum Publications, 1978

2. Frank J: Persuasion and Healing—A Comparative Study of Psychotherapy. Baltimore: The Johns Hopkins Press, 1961

3. Strupp H: Toward a reformulation of the psychotherapeutic influence. Int J Psychoanal 11:263-365, 1973

4. Ferenczi S: The further development of an active therapy in psychoanalysis, in Further Contributions to the Theory and Technique of Psychoanalysis. London, Hogarth Press, 1950

5. Alexander F, French TM: Psychoanalytic Therapy. New York, Ronald Press, 1946

6. Murphy WF: The Tactics of Psychotherapy. New York, International Universities Press, 1965

7. Malan D: The Frontiers of Brief Psychotherapy. New York, Plenum Medical Book Co., 1976

8. Mann J: Time-Limited Psychotherapy. Cambridge, Harvard University Press, 1973

9. Sifneos P: Short-Term Dynamic Psychotherapy: Evaluation and Technique. New York, Plenum Medical Book Co., 1979

10. Hartmann H: Ego Psychology and the Problem of Adaptation. Translated by Rapaport D. New York, International Universities Press, 1958

11. Diagnostic and Statistical Manual of Mental Disorders (Third Edition). Washington, D.C., American Psychiatric Association, 1980

12. Reich W: Character Analysis (Third Edition). New York, Noonday Press, 1949

13. Beck AT: Cognitive therapy: nature and relationship to behavior therapy. Behav Res Ther 1:184-200, 1970

14. Flegenheimer WV: Techniques of Brief Psychotherapy. New York, Jason Aronson, 1982

15. Gill M: Analysis of Transference, vol. I. New York, International Universities Press, 1982

16. Strachey J: The nature of the therapeutic action of psychoanalysis. Int J Psychoanal 15:127-159, 1934

4

The Impact of Short-Term Dynamic Psychotherapy on Psychoanalytic Psychotherapy

Victor Goldin, M.D.
Arnold Winston, M.D.

4

The Impact of Short-Term Dynamic Psychotherapy on Psychoanalytic Psychotherapy

Psychoanalysis had a double impact on psychiatry in the years after World War II. It bestowed a portion of its legacy on those therapists who received psychoanalytic training and embarked on a style of practice guided by orthodox Freudian precepts; and another portion, more widely diffused but less intensely concentrated, on those therapists who, though not psychoanalysts, found their practices molded by exposure to Freudian thought that pervaded contemporary psychiatry.

Four decades later, it may be anticipated that the increasing popularity of short-term dynamic psychotherapy will similarly generate both a community of orthodox practitioners and a wave of influence that will affect most other psychoanalytic therapists. In hazarding this speculation, we hope not to sound like the apostles of a new religion informing the pagans that their beliefs and customs are now obsolete. Rather, the confidence we have in the spreading influence of short-term dynamic psychotherapy stems from a sense that this therapy is part of a broader consensus among dynamic psychotherapists as they move toward a new definition of the therapeutic process. It is, at any rate, for future historians of psychiatry to locate the ultimate impact of short-term dynamic psychotherapy.

While a number of publications (1-4) have presented the

techniques of the leaders in the field, this chapter seeks to anticipate the nature of short-term dynamic psychotherapy's influence on psychoanalytic psychotherapists in general.

The gradual introduction, since 1980, of the teaching and practice of short-term dynamic psychotherapy at Beth Israel Medical Center in New York City has colored the practice of the traditional psychotherapists in contact with the core group. For our purposes, without denying the differences among the various "schools" of short-term dynamic psychotherapy, what emerges most clearly is the psychoanalytic heritage they share (1,2,4,5). The development of short-term dynamic psychotherapy from psychoanalysis recalls the growth of psychoanalytic therapy from its psychoanalytic roots. This kinship suggests that the engrafting of short-term dynamic psychotherapy might well strengthen the body of psychotherapy. This issue of integration of psychoanalytic psychotherapy and short-term dynamic psychotherapy has not been vigorously addressed.

The void thus created helps to promote the impression that practitioners of traditional psychotherapy and psychoanalysis might find their techniques weakened by exposure to those of short-term dynamic psychotherapy. This fear of dilution was with us as we introduced short-term dynamic psychotherapy into the repertoire of our department. The opposite seems to have occurred.

We have reported elsewhere on the effects of the introduction of short-term dynamic psychotherapy on residency training (6). We now turn our attention to a group of more advanced psychotherapists to assess the changes in their practice brought about by exposure to an environment heavily colored by the techniques of short-term dynamic psychotherapy.

Before proceeding to gauge the effects of short-term dynamic psychotherapy on psychoanalytic psychotherapy, we note elements basic to both. Psychoanalytic psychotherapy, with its analytic underpinnings, aims in large measure at uncovering psychic conflict. This characteristic it clearly shares with short-term dynamic psychotherapy. Those readers who seek greater familiarity with the "schools" of short-term dynamic psychotherapy are referred to Flengenheimer's concise summary (5). It is, however, the supportive elements interwoven with the procedures designed primarily to promote insight that give psychoanalytic psychotherapy its richness, complexity, and usefulness. There is a common misconception that views short-term dynamic psychotherapy, because of its directness, as lacking in supportive qualities. This is decidedly not the case. We believe Alexander (7) had a clearer view when he wrote, "It is customary to divide psychotherapeutic procedures into two categories: the supportive and uncovering procedures. It must be born in mind, however, that supportive measures knowingly or inadvertently are used in all forms of psychotherapy, and conversely some degree of insight is rarely absent from any sound psychotherapeutic approach" (p. 280).

We will postpone further inquiry into the questions of what constitutes support, and what are the kinds of support, in short-term dynamic psychotherapy. At this point in our efforts to understand the effects of short-term dynamic psychotherapy on dynamic psychotherapy, we only wish to note that in spite of its dedication to uncovering, focused inquiry, and confrontation, supportive elements are by no means absent from this technique. In this we agree with the basic premises of Rogers (8) when he suggested that the patient's feeling of trust in the therapist and belief that the therapist understands him are critical. Equally congenial is Enelow's (9) suggestion that the therapist's communication of liking the patient is inherently supportive. This is related to empathy and its role in both supportive and exploratory psychotherapy. It is also clear that abreaction, with its expression of powerful feelings in the presence of a nonjudgmental therapist, supports the patient's ego.

We will now turn to the major focus of this chapter. We will illustrate the ways in which the short-term dynamic psychotherapist functions in the evaluation of a patient, and the ways in which he or she handles those two analytic cornerstones, resistance and transference. Once this is clear, we will comment on the effects on traditional psychotherapists who are exposed to this work.

EVALUATION

The initial evaluation of a patient for short-term dynamic psychotherapy is a major undertaking and has great significance. It is a vigorous, sometimes lengthy process. Evaluation interviews conducted at the Beth Israel Medical Center for Training and Research in Short-Term Dynamic Psychotherapy are characterized by:

1. Great activity on the part of the interviewer.

2. Efforts directed at obtaining precise, detailed and meaningful information.

3. A thorough inventory of areas of disturbance.

4. Testing of motivation for change.

5. The evocation of significant feelings.

6. Tests of impulse control.

7. Assessments of psychological mindedness.

8. A rich description of interpersonal interaction with one or more significant persons in the patient's current life.

9. Operations designed to focus the patient's attention on his or her feelings toward the interviewer.

10. Obtaining other information customarily sought in a psychiatric interview, such as: a description and dynamic understanding of the family of origin; work and school history; social history; sexual history, including fantasy life at different stages of development; marital history; depression (degree and kind; suicide potential); anxiety (degree and kind; disorganizing effects of anxiety); history of significant physical and mental illness and treatments.

All of the interviews are videotaped, as are most short-term dynamic psychotherapy sessions. The reader is asked to imagine the effect that viewing these interviews has on a traditional psychoanalytic psychotherapist.

What follows is an example illustrative of short-term dynamic therapists' work. This is a significantly edited and condensed version of a segment of an interview that actually took 15 minutes.

Case Example

The patient is a 32-year-old, self-referred biochemist. He is carefully and conservatively dressed. Seven minutes have elapsed since he came into the office. In that time he has, in a controlled and mechanical manner, commented on his dissatisfaction with his life. He is particularly concerned that he is not married, and is worried because he never seems to meet the right women. He hints that he has sexual difficulty with "my present woman friend." The therapist, sensing the monotony of the interview up to this point, has just asked for her name.

P: As I was saying, I have this general sense—
T: With Jane?
P: Yes, a discontented—
T: Discontented?
P: Yes its a global feeling when I'm with her.
T: Now a global feeling.
P: Yes a global feeling.
T: What do you mean?
P: As I was saying a general sense.
T: That is very vague.
P: I'm trying to clarify it.
T: But, you remain vague.
P: I guess that's one of my problems.
T: Now guessing, still vague.
P: I can't pin it down.
T: Now you become helpless.
P: I didn't say I was helpless.
T: You act helpless.
P: Helpless is your word.
T: You come in and you're helpless to tell me your problems.
P: It's hard to be more specific (head slumps slightly forward)
T: So now you go limp.
P: I don't seem to be getting anyplace. (voice rising slightly)
T: Again, helpless.
P: One can't just immediately put his finger on things. (the tone is rising and there is slight sarcastic underscoring of "immediately")
T: We are talking of you.
P: OK, I can't immediately put my finger where you want. (Sounding annoyed) It's damn difficult given this situation and all the pressure.
T: Again, helpless.
P: I sure don't know what you want. (muscles in jaw tighten, averts gaze)

T: You look away.
P: (Looks back toward therapist and then again, averts eyes)
T: Again, do you notice, you look away.
P: OK. (glares at therapist)
T: (Noting patient's now clenched fists) You have some feelings.
P: I'm a little annoyed.
T: A little.
P: I'm annoyed.
T: You say annoyed; how do you feel?
P: Frustrated and annoyed.
T: Your fists are clenched.
P: I'm angry.
T: You're angry toward me.
P: Yes, frustrated and angry.
T: How do you feel?
P: You don't make things easier—I thought psychiatrists helped people.
T: How do you experience the anger?
P: I don't know.
T: Again, helpless.
P: Anger is anger.
T: Anger is a word. The anger, how do you feel it?
P: I feel hot all over.
T: Hot.
P: Hot! Hot and like I'm going to explode.
T: Like you're going to explode toward me?
P: Yeah, I feel I could explode all over you.
T: You would do what to me?
P: I'd like to cream you.
T: Cream me?
P: Haul off, cream you, and then walk out.

The last statement showed considerable rise in emotional tone. The therapist linked this with feelings toward Jane. The patient was now able to note that angry feelings lay just underneath his generally discontented feelings. This was especially evident when they were sexually involved. Jane seemed to him very demanding ("She wants me to touch just the right place") and is not very helpful ("She hints but doesn't really let me know what she wants"). As he continues to explore his feelings of frustration and anger toward Jane, he recognizes the desire to "do something to her." Further exploration revealed that the "do something to her" becomes having an ejaculation extra-vaginally (cream all over her) and then go to sleep (walk out).

Fifteen minutes further into the interview the patient is discussing his surrogate mother, Aunt Selma (his own mother was often in the hospital). He spoke of her demandingness and of her failure to instruct him and help him. He had a sense of general uneasiness with her. His anger with Aunt Selma was well controlled because he feared abandonment.

Many traditional psychotherapists, upon first witnessing such a confrontational interview, complain that the patient is being badgered. Psychotherapists are concerned, appropriately, about this procedure harming patients. They are somewhat reassured when the evaluator explains that he or she recognizes the stress placed on the patient, and is alert for signs of disorganization or fragmentation. If this occurs, the interviewer is always prepared to shift to a less confrontational, more supportive style. In time, most traditional therapists come to appreciate the skill of the evaluators in their ability to maintain pressure as long as necessary, and to ease off only if the patient is in danger. Discomfort to either patient or therapist is not necessarily dangerous.

Attitudes of traditional psychoanalytic therapists change after exposure to a number of such evaluations. Talk of the interviewer badgering the patient fades away. Over time the staff observing these interviews notes that patients do not suffer psychotic decompensations or prolonged depressions.

The conclusion of the above interview 2¾ hours later comes as a pleasant surprise to many observers. The interview has been punctuated several times by intense interactions. The patient and the therapist have both worked hard. The patient seems somewhat elated. His manner has changed. He is less detached, he holds his body less rigidly. He seems more in touch with his feelings and with the therapist.

T: How do you feel about what went on here today?
P: I was really impressed.
T: Impressed?
P: I was surprised and pleased so much came out.
T: Surprised about what?
P: I didn't realize I had so much anger and sadness in me. (At points the patient had wept, particularly when he talked of his inability to get close to his father.)

T: You recognized new genuine feelings.
P: Yes—they were genuine all right.
T: How do you feel toward me?
P: I got pretty sore at you at times, but you really helped.
T: Do you think if you continued in therapy as we have been doing this morning, it would be helpful to you?
P: I sure think so. I'd like to try.

Traditional psychotherapists report that their own evaluations are modified by watching these taped interviews. They become more active, more courageous in pursuing feelings, appreciably more specific and concrete in delineating chief complaints, and generally more in control of the interview. None of the therapists who noted these changes felt that such exposure confused their technique or made them less effective. A few reported that viewing the tapes made little or no difference in their functioning. Most therapists also noted that if they did not continue to observe the short-term dynamic psychotherapy evaluation process they would drift back, sooner or later, toward their previous, less active, less focused style.

RESISTANCE

There can be no understanding of the psychotherapies based on psychoanalytic principles without reference to resistance. In his 50 years of developing theory and technique, Freud constantly returned to this critical element. His papers touching on the subject lead from Studies on Hysteria (10), Interpretation of Dreams (11), Inhibitions, Symptoms and Anxiety (12), to Analysis, Terminable and Interminable (13). Freud (14) had termed resistance a cornerstone of his theory. No one has found reason to dispute that appellation. The varieties of resistances are potentially without limit. The classification and techniques for analyzing resistances occupies a considerable part of Greenson's (15) standard work.

Of the many techniques used by short-term dynamic psychotherapists to overcome resistance, we limit our illustrations to three: therapist activity, the use of detailing, and thwarting regression. These few are chosen because they readily lend themselves to integration into the armamentarium of dynamic psychotherapists. The role of transference in overcoming resistance is of the utmost importance. This is addressed later in this Chapter.

Activity on the Part of the Therapist

The silent analyst listening with "even hovering attention" is an image that has confounded the performance of many psychoanalytic psychotherapists. While much of what Freud recommended has been readily adopted, his practice in regard to activity has suffered a different fate. At least one of his analysands saw him as quite active. Kanzer (16) criticized Freud as too active. Greenson (15) warned "too much activity may interfere with the patients' ability for being active and gratify his passive wishes."

During the third psychotherapy session, the patient described earlier noted that he discussed Jane at length with several of his friends. The details of what he told them came like a flood and seemed likely to overwhelm and inundate the hour. Seizing the moment, the short-term dynamic therapist said:

T: You ask everyone's opinion of Jane.
P: Not everyone.
T: But you seem to ask everyone about Jane.
P: Well . . . I like to have feedback.
T: You need continuous feedback.
P: It's very important to me, what my friends think.
T: It seems their approval is very important to you.
P: Now that you say it, yes, I guess so.
T: You guess.
P: No, I'm sure it's so.
T: Now with John, you were telling me what you told him about Jane at lunch.
P: Yes.
T: Let's look at that in greater detail.
P: We had lunch and I brought it up—Jane—pros and cons.
T: Where were you having lunch?
P: We met and brown bagged it at Citicorp, yesterday.
T: You were at Citicorp and what was happening?
P: I bought coffee to be able to use one of those tables near the Espresso place.
T: What exactly went on with you and John in discussing Jane?

P: I knew before we met that I'd tell him about her. Almost as soon as we sat down I turned the conversation around.

T: What exactly did you tell him?

P: Well I started out generally describing our relationship.

T: You say generally, but it was only yesterday. Can't you be more specific? Is your memory bad?

P: I told John she demanded a lot.

T: Yes.

P: I told him she was demanding.

T: Yes, but what did you really say?

P: I've known John since we were in college together.

T: You haven't told me what you really said.

P: We kidded around a bit and then I told him she wasn't good in bed.

T: You were sitting at one of those little tables in Citicorp, talking to John, you can remember the moment very clearly, it was just yesterday. What did you say exactly?

P: I'm not proud of what I said.

T: We are not talking proud.

P: I guess I wanted him—to enjoy that—to be on my side—a kind of team with me.

T: What did you say?

P: His approval was important.

T: Have you noticed you aren't telling me what you said?

P: (Looking sheepish) I told him she made love like a dead fish.

The patient said he felt that he had betrayed Jane to win John's approval and affection. He then remembered a dream:

It was a narrow crooked street—European—set somehow on Fifth Avenue (where he now lives). His association (provoked by the therapist's active questioning) led to a memory of his going to Europe with his father and Aunt Selma. He was very small. He had made a joke about his mother (she was then home or in the hospital). His father seemed to think it was funny.

In this segment, the therapist says a great deal, but he does not stop the patient's flow nor does it appear that he gratifies his patient's passivity. Discussions with traditional therapists have led us to conclude that these therapists are actually more active in their psychotherapy than they care to admit publicly. Watching the work of short-term dynamic therapists seems to have a liberalizing effect. They concentrate more directly on what they are doing in therapy. Viewing the tapes helps other therapists report more accurately and more clearly on their own, as opposed to their patients', activity.

The Use of Detail

Several of the above vignettes are in themselves examples of the use of details. When they find themselves in emotionally loaded territory, short-term dynamic psychotherapists often heighten the impact by honing in on details.

The death of this patient's father, when he was eight, was a grievous loss. He had not been told by Aunt Selma, his mother, or his grandmother, that his father had angina. The day of his father's death had already been approached in the initial interview. Now in the sixth session it came up again.

T: Just what were you doing that day?
P: I don't know. I was only seven or eight.
T: You remember where you lived?
P: Oh yes, the house on Ryder Road.
T: Tell me about your father's death.
P: I know I was home. Not in school.
T: How do you know that?
P: It must have been Saturday. I was across the street at the G's. I remember they got a phone call and told me I should go home, but it was only 11:30, not even time for lunch. I went home. I walked on the porch. That's the way I always did. I liked to rock on the step. It was rotting, sort of, and it had a bounce to it.
T: You came up onto the porch and then what? Who was there?
P: Aunt Selma. She had been crying I guess. She looked odd and said, "Your father has taken a trip." My grandmother looked funny too. Then they said I should go back and play. I asked about the trip, but no one said anything.
T: What did you do?
P: I went back across the street to play. Frankie had a game of Clue and I played with him and his sister. I went home after awhile.
T: What happened exactly?
P: No. I didn't go home really. My grandmother took me to her house. I tried to ask about the trip and all, but nobody would say anything. My grandfather came home and I was always scared around him. I remember that meal. It was very quiet.
T: Did you sleep at your grandparents?

P: No, I didn't have my pajamas. When I got back to my house, my grown-up cousin was leaving.

T: Did you go to bed?

P: Yes.

T: Where did you sleep?

P: I had a room at the head of the stairs.

T: Did you have any routine at bedtime?

P: What do you mean, routine?

T: What did you do before you went to sleep? Specifically, in detail, I mean when you were seven or eight.

P: I always lined up my toy cars in parallel rows. I remember I couldn't sleep if I didn't do that.

T: You remember lining up your cars. You can visualize that. You look as if your eyes are watering.

P: (Sighing) Then I'd go kiss him goodnight.

T: Tell me just what you did.

P: (Now sobbing) I'd put on my bunny slippers and run downstairs and kiss Daddy goodnight.

T: And that night?

P: My grandmother came up and said my father had gone on a trip. (Crying clearly now)

T. You're crying.

P. (Through the tears) He always said he'd die if I didn't kiss him goodnight. (Continues with sobs) For years after that I'd see him in heaven with a suitcase. I thought he'd gone on a trip.

The short-term dynamic psychotherapists' asking detailed questions seems to be one technique that most traditional psychotherapists easily adopt. It fits comfortably into the repertoire of traditional psychotherapists. They find it particularly helpful in working with pathological mourning (see Chapter Two of this monograph).

Thwarting Regression

The short-term dynamic psychotherapist cannot afford to let a patient regress and then analyze the regression. Evidence of movement to a less mature position needs to be interpreted as soon as it is detected.

In the 12th session, facing up to his dissatisfaction at work, our patient reported having acted incompetently with his boss. He feared to cut loose from a benevolent father figure, and recapitulated this behavior with his therapist.

P: I don't know what to talk about today.
T: Go on.
P: I just can't seem to think of anything that matters.
T: Have you noticed that you come in and act helpless?
P: I can't be blamed, I just don't have any thoughts.
T: You suddenly stop thinking? Can we look at that?
P: I don't have any thoughts.
T: Let's look at that.
P: I told you—I don't have any clear thoughts.
T: So, if you continue to have no thoughts, what will happen?
P: I don't know what you mean.
T: What will happen to you?
P: What will happen to me?
T: You act puzzled and dull.
P: I don't know what you are getting at.
T: If you continue to have no thoughts, then what will happen here in your therapy?
P: Well, we won't make any progress.
T: And if your therapy is unsuccessful what will happen to you?
P: I guess I will just go on.
T: Right. You will continue with a life that is unsatisfactory.
P: Mmmm.
T: And the problems you came in here with and the suffering will continue.
P: You're right—I guess.
T: You say I guess. But you're the one that will be stuck with what you call "a lousy job with a good boss." You are the one who will live and die without a close relationship with a woman. So what are we going to do about this?

The patient then went on to talk about his dissatisfaction at work and his fury with his boss.

The patient, prodded by the therapist from time to time (an appeal to the healthy part of the ego), will move "up the ladder," and motivation will increase. Regression, which included a cognitive retreat to helplessness and dullness, was arrested and reversed by the end of the hour. The patient had worked on his early fears of independence in a home which seemed, at best, tentative. Regression, in some patients, takes the form of tears. Once the therapist ascertains that this is defensive, it is handled in the same manner as cognitive regression, through interpretation.

Transference

The development and subsequent resolution of the transference neurosis has been the vehicle of emotional growth and resolution of conflict in classical analysis. Psychoanalytic psychotherapies have borrowed this most important concept. The setting of psychoanalytic psychotherapy, however, does not lend itself as easily as does analysis to the fullest development of transference distortions. There is the matter of frequency. Patients seeing an analyst four and five times a week are more likely to develop a full blown transference neurosis. The analyst encourages free association and strives to present a blank screen. The couch, with the analyst out of site, plays a part. Psychoanalytic psychotherapists can count on only a partial development of a transference neurosis. As a consequence, the resolution of the transference neurosis in psychoanalytic psychotherapies is also less clear.

The position of the short-term dynamic psychotherapist is different. Short-term dynamic psychotherapy does not encourage the development of a regressive transference neurosis. The time involved in this process would make therapy of 20 to 40 weeks impossible. Short-term dynamic psychotherapists claim successful resolution of a wide variety of clinical conditions without resort to this basic technical maneuver. The results reported by these therapists are now being put through vigorous research evaluation. Preliminary data suggest that their methods, used with selected patients, have achieved enduring changes.

It is hard to discern any clear-cut impact that this fundamental difference in theory might have on practicing psychoanalytically oriented psychotherapists who have been exposed to the work of short-term dynamic psychotherapists. This may be so because while many psychotherapists talk about transference neurosis, they don't have the same commitment to the concept that their analytic colleagues do. At least we have found few therapists who document the development of transference neurosis and demonstrate that its working through has been a truly integral part of successful therapy.

It is, rather, in the psychoanalytic literature that there seems to be movement and change. Gill (17) has argued for early interpretations of the transference. He suggests that Freud's precept that transference only be interpreted when it is a resistance needs to be taken more literally and more broadly. In his view, transference often functions as a resistance from the beginning. Psychoanalytic psychotherapists who watch the work of short-term dynamic psychotherapists are more receptive to Gill's broader view of transference. He suggests that the relationship and interactions with the therapist have, from the outset, the coloration of earlier significant relationships. He argues that the projection of these internalized objects onto the therapist is constantly taking place. The short-term dynamic psychotherapist shares a similar position. Constant attention to and interpretation of the transference will prevent the development of a transference neurosis. Malan (18) believes that the kind of interpretation and linkages in the illustration that follows are indicative of successful therapy. Our patient returned again to his complaint about the therapist. Once more in the 18th session, as in the initial evaluation, he began:

P: I have an uneasy sense today.

T: An uneasy sense?

P: Yes. I don't feel comfortable with you.

T: How do you feel?

P: I'm tense, that's all.

T: Tense? What are you feeling?

P: You seem angry. You walked down the hall briskly, like you were preoccupied.

T: And you felt?

P: Alone, lost a little—scared I guess.

T: What else?

P: I was all tense when I came in today. I tried to find some way to make you smile. I keep having the feeling that you didn't want to see me today. I found myself trying to entertain.

T: That's like what in your past?

P: That's exactly how I always felt with Aunt Selma. I just had exactly the same feeling.

T: You felt the same way with me that you did with Aunt Selma?

P: Exactly. The circumstances. Age different, of course, but I felt just

> the same. Small, unwanted, alone. It's uncanny—but I really felt just like I did when I was five.
>
> During the remainder of this session, the therapist linked similar feelings to the patient's woman friend, Jane. The therapist guided the patient back and forth along a triangle that linked a past figure (Aunt Selma) to a current figure (Jane) and to the therapist.

One of our traditionally oriented psychotherapists viewing this tape likened it to a spider spinning a web—back and forth, catching first the transference figure, then the past figure (Aunt Selma), then the current figure (Jane). The emotional threads were similar and he said, "It made a good tight package." It is too early in the continuing discussion about broadening the concepts of transference and the potential advantage of early interpretation of transference to know if Gill's views will fall by the wayside or will signal a substantial change in the way the concept of transference is used in psychoanalysis and psychotherapy in the future.

CONCLUSION

Short-term dynamic psychotherapy informs psychoanalytic psychotherapy. Coexisting, they cannot help but modify each other. We have addressed aspects of short-term dynamic psychotherapy as seen in evaluation, and worked with resistance and transference, and suggested how they "rub off" onto the traditional psychoanalytic psychotherapist.

We hope that this report of our observations within one department of psychiatry will encourage others to look at additional examples of the confluence of dynamic psychotherapeutic techniques. We trust that parochial aims, advancing the truth of one technique over the other, will not cloud understanding of the direction and continuing movement of psychotherapy as practiced by most American psychiatrists.

References

1. Davanloo H: Basic Principles and Techniques in Short-Term Dynamic Psychotherapy. New York, Spectrum Publications, 1978

2. Malan D: The Frontiers of Brief Psychiatry. New York, Plenum Medical Book Company, 1976

3. Mann J: Time-Limited Psychotherapy. Cambridge, Harvard University Press, 1973

4. Sifneos P: Short-Term Dynamic Psychotherapy: Evaluation and Technique. New York, Plenum Medical Book Company, 1979

5. Flegenheimer WV: Techniques of Brief Psychotherapy. New York, Jason Aronson, 1982

6. Goldin V, Said T, Luis A, et al: Impact of Short-Term Focal Therapy on Residents. American Psychiatric Association 137th Annual Meeting, Syllabus and Scientific Proceedings, Los Angeles, May, 1984

7. Alexander F: The Scope of Psychoanalysis. New York, Basic Books, 1961

8. Rogers CR: The characteristics of a helping relationship, in Contemporary Psychotherapies. Edited by Stein MJ. New York, Free Press of Glencoe, 1962

9. Enelow AJ: Elements of Psychotherapy. New York, Oxford University Press, 1977

10. Breuer J, Freud S: Studies on hysteria (1893-1895), in Complete Psychological Works, Standard Edition, vol. 2. Translated and edited by Strachey J. London, Hogarth Press, 1955

11. Freud S: The interpretation of dreams (1900), in Complete Psychological Works, Standard Edition, vols. 4, 5. Translated and edited by Strachey J. London, Hogarth Press, 1953

12. Freud S: Inhibitions, symptoms and anxiety (1925-1926), in Com-

plete Psychological Works, Standard Edition, vol. 20. Translated and edited by Strachey J. London, Hogarth Press, 1959

13. Freud S: Analysis, terminable and interminable (1937), in Complete Psychological Works, Standard Edition, vol. 23. Translated and edited by Strachey J. London, Hogarth Press, 1923

14. Freud S: Freud's psychoanalytic procedure (1904 [1903]), in Complete Psychological Works, Standard Edition, vol. 7. Translated and edited by Strachey J. London, Hogarth Press, 1953

15. Greenson R: The Technique and Practice of Psychoanalysis, vol. 1. New York, International Universities Press, 1967

16. Kanzer M: The transference neurosis of the Rat Man. Psychoanal Q 21:181-189, 1952

17. Gill MM, Muslin HL: Early interpretation of transference. J Am Psychoanal Assoc 24:779-794, 1976

18. Malan DH: A Study of Brief Psychotherapy. New York, Plenum Press, 1963

5

Research Issues in Short-Term Dynamic Psychotherapies: An Overview

Manuel Trujillo, M.D.
Leigh McCullough, Ph.D.

5

Research Issues in Short-Term Dynamic Psychotherapies: An Overview

This chapter will briefly review recent clinical and methodological advances that have sparked renewed interest in psychotherapy research, before going on to describing Beth Israel Medical Center's study on the process and outcome of short-term dynamic psychotherapy on personality disorders.

During the last three decades the field of psychotherapy research has struggled with three fundamental questions:

1. Is psychotherapy effective?
2. If so, are the effects specific?
3. What is the scientific and clinical status of psychodynamic psychotherapy?

Is Psychotherapy Effective?

In 1952, reporting on 19 studies covering more than 7,000 patients and dealing both in psychoanalytic and "eclectic cases," Eysenck (1) reached a conclusion that will trouble the psychoanalytic community for years to come. "These data fail to prove that psychotherapy, Freudian or otherwise, facilitates the recovery of neurotic patients. They show that roughly two-thirds of a group of neurotic patients will recover or improve within about two years of the onset of their illness, whether they are treated by means of psychotherapy or not" (p. 323). With characteristic prescience he went on to predict that this argument would not be easily accepted by the psychotherapeutic community. Eysenck's challenge stimulated a torrent of psychotherapy studies; and a very high percentage of the 400 studies reviewed by Smith et al (2) quote Eysenck's original study.

If Eysenck fired the opening salvo with the question, "Is psychotherapy effective?", Smith et al (2), with their landmark study, provided sufficient evidence to definitively close the effectiveness question.

In a study characterized by methodological innovations, they showed that "the average person receiving treatment is better off than 80 percent of untreated control." They indicated that improvement in self-esteem and in symptoms such as anxiety are considerably larger than changes in personal, school, and work functioning. The average largest effect size goes to systematic desensitization, with psychodynamic psychotherapies occupying an intermediate position in the effectiveness spectrum.

A notable feature of the study is its comprehensiveness: out of almost 1,000 studies examined, 500 were selected and 375 fully analyzed, thus establishing a justifiable claim to generalizability of results.

IF SO, ARE THE EFFECTS SPECIFIC?

The appropriate paradigmatic studies include those of Frank (3) and Strupp (4), arguing for the importance of nonspecific factors, and Weissman's (5) and Beck's (6) studies supporting the specificity of therapeutic effects and techniques. Frank, in a series of outcome studies of a variety of individual and group therapies of six months' average duration, demonstrated comparable improvement in symptoms, subjective discomfort, and social ineffectiveness, at termination and two years later. Although he failed to describe his techniques in detail (thus earning the potential criticism that, of course, poorly specified techniques lead to nonspecific results) he proved that very different forms of psychotherapy can lead to positive effects and measurable changes. Since these changes cannot be ascribed to specific therapeutic techniques, they are accounted for by two mechanisms: *1.* the potentiation and activation of the patient's favorable expectations; and 2. the mobilization of latent affects, which may create more favorable conditions for assessing adaptive attitudes.

Strupp (7), in a series of reports coming out of the Vanderbilt Psychotherapy Study, could not demonstrate any effect of the therapist on outcome. Personable college professors of English performed as well as trained therapists did in the short-term treatment of college students suffering from anxiety, depression, and social isolation. However, in this study, techniques were not specified in advance and the treatment was not closely monitored. This may lead to an unfocused therapy, which is difficult to distinguish from that of sympathetic and experienced people with common sense.

On the other side of the specificity argument, the studies of Weissman (5) and Beck (6) represent powerful paradigms of "state of the art" psychotherapy studies. They include carefully defined therapeutic ingredients applied under monitored conditions to homogeneous groups of patients. Based on the premise that depression is basically a problem of cognition—the content of thinking is disturbed—Beck and colleagues (8) have developed a short-term (12 to 20 weeks) therapy. Traditional behavioral and cognitive techniques are employed, which encourage the patient to test and correct against reality excessively negative views of the self, the world, and the future. In a series of studies of efficacy, cognitive treatment has shown significant superiority over a variety of controls, including medication (imipramine) in patients suffering from depression (see Table 1). Similar findings are claimed by Weissman (5) for interpersonal psychotherapy, another form of short-term therapy developed for depression.

Based on the assumption that depression occurs in an interpersonal context, interpersonal therapy (IPT) focuses on recent interpersonal experiences by concentrating on one of four problem areas characteristic of depression: abnormal grief; interpersonal disputes; role transition; or interpersonal deficits.

These studies by Weissman (5) and Beck (6) represent the state of the art of well designed treatment studies because they include:

1. clearly specified techniques where application is guided by comprehensive treatment manuals and monitored by way of content analysis of therapy sessions;
2. homogeneous sample of patients;
3. standardized outcome measurements sampling multiple areas of patient functioning.

A major limitation of these studies is the relatively infrequent use of these techniques in actual practice, which limits their general applicability. Therefore the notion, "specific techniques lead to specific outcomes" cannot be expanded to psychoanalytically based psychotherapy, which is still widely practiced in the field. This issue leads us to our third question.

What is the Scientific and Clinical Status of Psychoanalytically Based Psychotherapy Today?

Sifneos (9, 10) has developed a form of psychodynamic psychotherapy—short-term anxiety-provoking psychotherapy (STAPP)—which he applies to patients suffering from anxiety, phobias, mild to moderate obsessive symptomatology, depression, and a variety of interpersonal problems. Patients are selected for Sifneos's therapy on the basis of clinical selection criteria, including the presence of motivation, average intelligence, psychological mindedness, and the ability to interact with the evaluator and others.

The patient must have an oedipal conflict as the basis of his or her symptomatology. Among his therapeutic techniques, Sifneos includes the selection of a focus, the use of anxiety-provoking confrontation, and active interpretation of material, as well as behavioral indicators of resistance.

Confrontation and clarification are also used to help the patient experience his transference feelings. "He (the therapist) bypasses character traits consistently, such as masochism, excessive passivity and dependence, which give rise to therapeutic complications" (p. 99).

Sifneos emphasizes the problem solving and learning nature of his psychotherapy. "The height of the treatment is characterized by the repeated efforts of the therapist to concentrate on the areas of unresolved conflict which underlie the patient's emotional problems, and to avoid the difficulties involving character traits which are considered to be more primitive" (p. 106). See Table 2 for a summary of the Sifneos approach.

Because of the presence of methodological limitations (which Sifneos himself readily admits), his studies can only be considered rich, well documented clinical and anecdotal descriptions of a form of psychotherapy that offers great potential if adequately tested.

In one of his studies, Sifneos reports on 21 patients who had an average of 20 sessions of short-term anxiety-provoking psychotherapy. They achieved moderate symptom improvement, as well as surprisingly lasting improvements in self-esteem, which were maintained at two- and four-year followup. The patients also reported an increase in their ability to deal with other people, and the project therapist described significant psychodynamic changes.

Malan (11, 12, 13), working in the Tavistock Clinic in London, has provided a number of ingenious, detailed, and well documented studies on the outcome of psychoanalytically based psychodynamic psychotherapy. Malan made elegant and significant contributions to help solve many methodological problems that have plagued outcome and process research on psychoanalytic psychotherapy. He reported that important and lasting changes, both symptomatic and psychodynamic, could be accomplished in patients suffering from severe psychopathology. Among many other contributions, he was able to show correlations between certain technical actions on the part of the therapist (that is, interpretations linking the therapist with significant figures in the patient's past) with a positive outcome at the end of the treatment. He also established that initial motivation as well as the maintenance of an agreed-upon psychodynamic focus correlated with success in brief psychotherapy.

The patients were selected for Malan's studies on the basis of clinical criteria, which included the following: the presence of a focus; the patient's demonstrated capacity to interact with the evaluator in a meaningful way; the patient's ability to establish good relationships with people in his or her past; and, most importantly, the response of the patient to active early interpretations of impulse and feelings ("trial interpretation"). Malan summarized his results as follows:

1. Relatively disturbed patients do respond to brief psychotherapy;
2. The more "radical" the technique the more favorable the outcome;
3. Motivation and focus are correlated with outcome;
4. The most important factor is linking transference-parent patterns;
5. The above findings constitute scientific validation of psychoanalytic principles (p. 54).

At the same time that Malan and Sifneos were engaged in their work, Davanloo, at the Montreal General Hospital of McGill University, produced three systematic clinical studies on the psychotherapeutic treatment of patients suffering from neuroses and character disorders (14, 15, 16). These studies, which can be described as sophisticated, clinical, non-controlled outcome evaluation studies, have become the basis for his technique of short-term dynamic psychotherapy. This is a psychoanalytically based form of psychotherapy which, Davanloo states, is specifically suited for the treatment of patients suffering from severe psychopathology, including stable and long-standing personality disorders. The patients treated by Davanloo were seen for an average of 20 sessions, and 40 percent had followups five to seven years later. He reports substantial clinical gains, which were maintained at termination and followup, with both baseline and outcome assessments performed by independent evaluators.

Davanloo (14) summarizes his technical principles as follows: "Common to all kinds of short-term dynamic psychotherapy is the activity of the therapist in the early utilization of transference and transference clarification and interpretation, maintaining the specific psychotherapeutic focus, the use of PT (past-transference) interpretation. The therapist actively works through any manifestation of resistance. Dream analysis and the analysis of defense are used. Therapy is terminated when evidence has been obtained that the central neurotic structure, which is at the core of all the patient's difficulties, has been resolved" (p. 14).

Other technical principles include the activity of the therapist in analyzing impulse, anxiety, and defense, and linking the transference with significant persons in the patient's past.

To summarize: Sifneos, Malan, and Davanloo, over the past two decades, have developed a range of short-term psychoanalytically based forms of psychotherapy. They have prepared the groundwork for significant research efforts by providing explicit criteria for the description and selection of the patient population for whom their psychotherapeutic techniques are applicable, and have delineated technical instructions and carefully documented clinical descriptions of the techniques and outcomes to be expected from their therapy.

The Beth Israel Medical Center Project

A clinical pilot study was started at Beth Israel Medical Center to test three hypotheses:

1. The ingredients of the therapeutic techniques proposed by Sifneos, Malan, and Davanloo can be studied under experimental conditions using measures sensitive to process and outcome changes. The requirements of blind and random assignments of patients to treatment conditions, which are standard for clinical trials in other disciplines, can also be applied to psychotherapy research.

2. Therapists can be trained to follow the prescriptions of treatment manuals, and can perform specific technical maneuvers in response to specific patient situations.

3. The active ingredients distilled from Malan's and Davanloo's

clinical work can be reliably coded by blind researchers from videotaped therapy sessions. Variables such as affect versus cognition, and level of use of the patient-therapist relationship, impact on the process and outcome of psychoanalytically based psychotherapy.

The Center has conducted a pilot study on the application of short-term psychotherapy techniques to patients suffering from a specific subset of personality disorders. At the present time a total of 14 women have been accepted. Their mean age is 36 years, ranging from 23 to 57. Six were single, four married, one separated, one divorced, and one widowed. Twelve of the 14 women have previously been in therapy. According to the *DSM-III* criteria, nine were diagnosed as mixed personality disorder, a majority with passive-aggressive features, three with avoidant personality disorder, one histrionic, and one compulsive. In terms of Axis I diagnosis, seven had dysthymic disorders, and the remainder had adjustment disorders with sexual, marital, or interpersonal difficulties.

The following instruments were used in the initial evaluations of these patients:

1. Diagnostic interview (semi-structured)
2. Personal and family history (semi-structured)
3. Brief adaptation-oriented psychotherapy (BAP) Assessment Form
4. Short-term dynamic psychotherapy (STDP) Assessment Form
5. Goal Attainment Scaling
6. Target Complaint Ratings (semi-structured)
7. Hopkins Symptom Check-List 90 Revised (SCL-90)
8. Health-Sickness Rating Scale
9. Structured and Scaled Interview to Assess Maladjustment (SSIAM)

Therapists. For each treatment condition there was a pool of psychiatrists, psychologists, and social workers, all of whom had a minimum of 12 months' training in brief psychotherapy. All therapists continued weekly seminars and supervision throughout the research project. The two therapist pools consisted of professionals with equivalent levels of training and experience. All psychotherapy sessions were videotaped in a standard format. All sessions were held weekly and lasted 50 minutes; fees were based on a sliding scale. Patients were held financially responsible for all sessions, including those missed for vacation.

Treatment Condition I. Brief adaptation-oriented psychotherapy (BAP; see Chapter Three of this monograph). This treatment condition includes therapeutic activities based on psychoanalytic principles, and reflects the state of the art of short-term psychoanalytically based psychotherapy in this country. The therapist is free to select a focus for his or her work, depending upon the patient's psychopathology. The focus involves uncovering the major maladaptive pattern of the patient. The aim is to provide a stabilizing framework for the patient's life, to help overcome interpersonal crises, to regain stability and/or emotional balance, and to develop a sense of self-esteem. Other goals may include the restoration or strengthening of defenses, as well as the promotion of a minimum of social and vocational adaptation.

Techniques include cognitive examination of intrapsychic and interpersonal conflicts. Catharsis may occur. The focus is on the ego, and efforts are not made to reach nuclear core pathology. Transference is interpreted only if it becomes a resistance, but no attempt is made to track it down and analyze it systematically. Severe character resistances are bypassed or dealt with by promoting cognitive insight.

Since this treatment has been developed for patients suffering from personality disorders, it will focus on these maladaptive, rigid and enduring patterns of perceiving, relating to, and thinking about the environment and the self, as well as behavior based on these patterns.

Treatment Condition II. Short-term dynamic psychotherapy (STDP; see Chapters One and Two of this monograph). This technique is based on the technique developed by Davanloo who, over the past 20 years, has been developing and perfecting a form of psychotherapy based on psychoanalytic principles that can effect changes in patients suffering from a variety of clinical syndromes and long-standing neurotic and personality disorders with severe psychopathology.

The differential ingredients of this technique as compared to the other four techniques of short-term psychotherapy include a high level of therapist activity, both the systematic confrontation and clarification of resistance (particularly of transference resistance), and the intensity and consistency of the psychotherapeutic work at the transference level.

As a result of this active psychotherapeutic process, affects are mobilized and worked through. They include sadness, anger, and anxiety, as well as warmth, personal closeness, and a desire for intimacy. These variables can be easily quantified and correlated with a variety of outcome dimensions, particularly those character features that most interfere with the functional adaptation of the patient. Data from our ongoing pilot study indicate that therapists can be trained to function within these parameters.

RESULTS OF PILOT STUDY

Of the 14 patients in the pilot study, ten have received mid-phase evaluations (at the 20th session). Five of these subjects were treated in the STDP short-term psychotherapy group and five were treated in the BAP short-term psychotherapy group. The four remaining subjects are now approaching their mid-phase evaluation. Of the ten patients who have received mid-phase evaluations, six have completed their 40th session, and the termination interviews are presently in progress. Two of the remaining subjects have dropped out of treatment, and two will complete therapy next month. No waiting list control data are yet available.

The pilot study results on outcomes are not yet available, but the results of two of our measures at mid-phase are indicative of their sensitivity to discriminate differences between groups. The measures we have analyzed so far are the Health Sickness Rating Scale (HSRS), which was done on each subject by an evaluator at intake and at mid-phase of therapy; and the Symptom Check List (SCL-90), which each subject filled out at intake and the mid-phase of therapy. These two measures are inversely related: the higher the HSRS score, the better the subject is functioning; the higher the SCL-90 score, the worse the subject is functioning in terms of severity of symptoms. Therefore, if both subject and evaluator agree on how the subject is doing, when one scale shows an increase, the other should show a decrease.

Figure 1 shows the mean ratings for the five subjects in the BAP short-term psychotherapy treatment group on each of the HSRS and SCL-90 scales, both at intake (solid lines) and at mid-phase (dotted line). The intake and mid-phase means appear to be virtually overlapping.

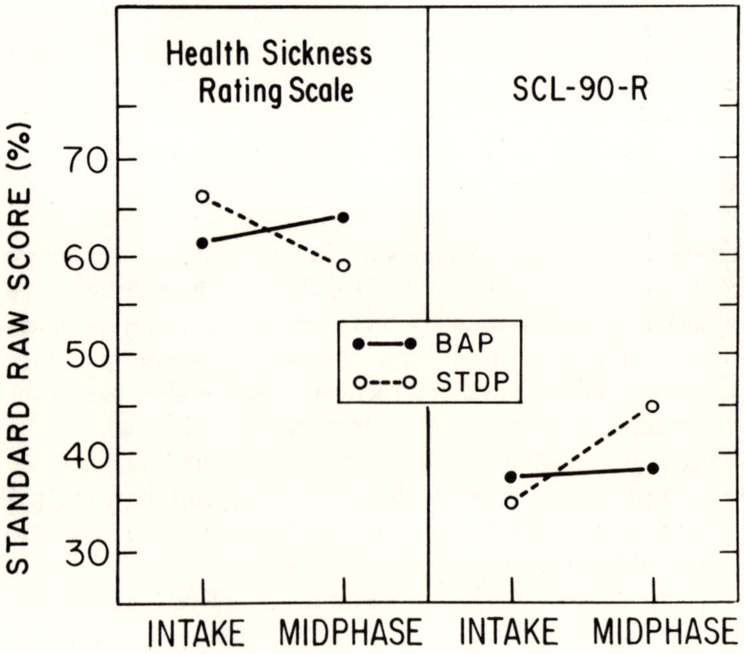

Figure 1. Variation in Patient Functioning on the HSRS and SCL-90 from Intake to Mid-phase for the BAP Group

Figure 2 shows the mean ratings for the five subjects in the STDP short-term psychotherapy group on each of the HSRS and SCL-90 scales, both at intake (solid circles) and at mid-phase (open circles). The intake and mid-phase means clearly separate out for all scales on each measure. At mid-phase the HSRS means are all lower (worse level of functioning), and SCL-90 means are all higher (worse level of functioning indicated by more symptoms). Thus, both evaluator and subject agree on how the subject is doing.

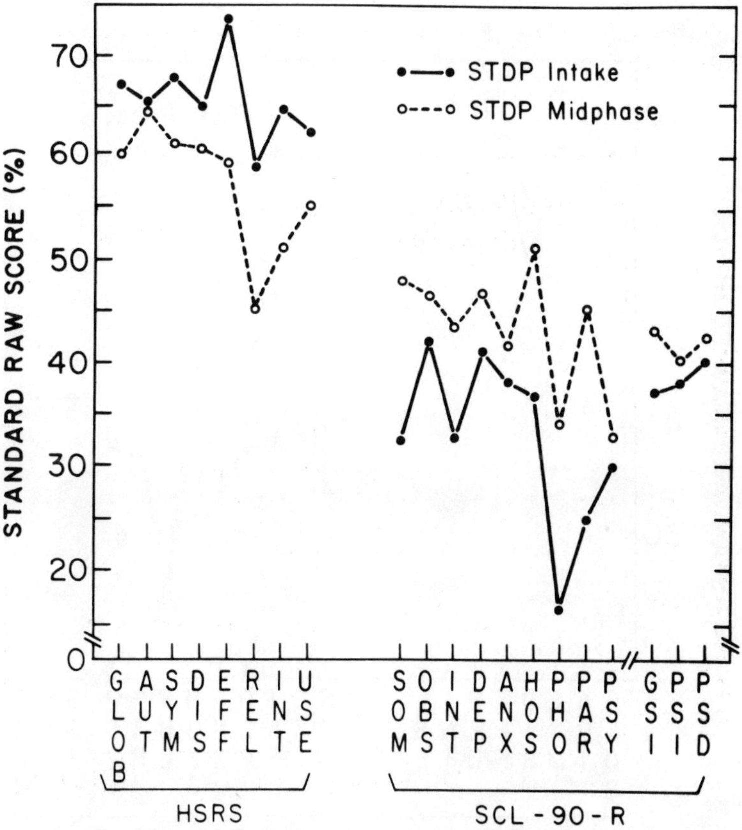

Figure 2. Variation in Patient Functioning on the HSRS and SCL-90 from Intake to Mid-phase on the STDP Group

Figure 3 shows the grand means of all HSRS and SCL-90 scales at intake and mid-phase for the BAP and for the STDP groups. The therapy by level of functioning (HSRS scale) and therapy by symptom (SCL-90 scale) interactions are clearly shown. Table 1 presents these grand mean values. Paired *t*-tests were used to assess the statistical significance of changes in these means from intake to mid-phase, since it is changes within subjects that the study addresses.

For the BAP therapy group, the SCL-90 means at intake and mid-phase are virtually identical (37.6 versus 38.42), and the increase in HSRS means (61.51 versus 64.43) is not statistically significant (t = 1.63; df = 4).

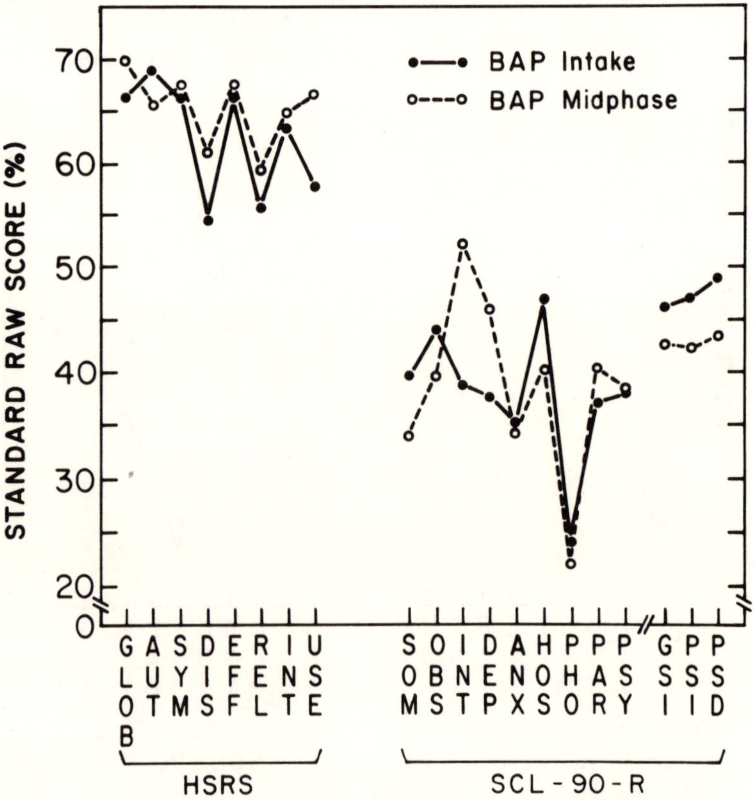

Figure 3. Comparison of the Two Treatment Groups at Intake and Mid-phase on the HSRS and SCL-90

Table 1. Cognitive Therapy of Depression

Theory:	The source of depression is a set of negative concepts. Correction of these concepts will eliminate depression.
Techniques:	1. Identify negative cognitions 2. Logical analysis and empirical testing to correct these distortions 3. Focus on target problems 4. Assignment of tasks to learn new ways of responding 5. Practice, in session and with homework
Successful outcomes:	The incorporation by the patient of many of the therapeutic techniques. A review of eight published reports of cognitive therapy showed significant superiority over controls. Patients ranged from mildly depressed college students to depressed hospital patients.

Reprinted from Beck AT, Ruch AJ, Shaw BF, et al. Cognitive Therapy of Depression. New York, Guilford Press, 1979. Reprinted by permission.

For the STDP therapy group, however, the SCL-90 means appear quite different at intake and at mid-phase (34.99 versus 45.29). Although this difference is ten times greater than for the BAP group, it does not reach statistical significance on a paired *t*-test (t = 1.86; df = 4). The HSRS means at intake and mid-phase not only show a large decrease (67.07 versus 58.76), but this difference is statistically significant (t = 2.83; df = 4; $p < .05$).

Thus, the HSRS and SCL-90 scales show an increase in symptoms and subjective distress at mid-phase in the STDP group, but the BAP group shows either no change or a slight decrease. This finding is supportive of our notion that the STDP psychotherapy is particularly effective in mobilizing affect, and shows that this process is differentially underway in the STDP group at mid-phase.

In summary, the above findings indicate: *1.* the HSRS and SCL-90 measures are capable of discriminating differential responses between the two treatment groups; and 2. that the therapist ratings (HSRS) corroborate the ratings of the patients (SCL-90), indicating the validity of the measures as indicative of patient functioning.

CODING OF VIDEOTAPED SESSIONS

During the past 12 months, extensive work has been performed in the development of a reliable system to code videotaped sessions. All sessions have been videotaped by the therapist and stored in the videotape library to be coded by the research assistants trained to a level of .80 reliability. The coding system, though based on extensive preliminary testing, still represents an early stage in the evolution of a coding system. Extensive research must be performed on every facet of this process before a truly standardized procedure can be established. However, preliminary analyses of interrater reliability have been performed, as well as analyses on the capability of this system to distinguish between two different treatment groups. These preliminary results are presented below.

Therapist Activity Variables

The variables chosen for therapist activity fall into two main categories. First are those standard techniques used by our therapists, which are also highly represented in the therapy process

Table 2. Sifneos's Short-Term Anxiety-Provoking Psychotherapy

Patient Selection:	1. Above average intelligence
	2. One meaningful relationship
	3. Emotional Crisis
	4. Able to express feelings and interact well with therapist
	5. Motivation for therapy
	6. Specific chief complaint
Techniques:	1. Early and repeated interpretation of resistance, ambivalence, and negative transference
	2. Deliberately provoking anxiety
	3. Use of examples in the transference
	4. Linking past patterns to transference behavior
Differs from Psychoanalysis in the Following:	1. Active avoidance of deep-seated characterological problems
	2. Avoidance of transference neurosis
	3. *Early termination*

literature; for example, Weiner (17). These include questions, clarifications, confrontations, interpretations, suggestions, and empathic comments. The second category of variables are those which differentiate our two experimental groups. These include therapists' questions that focus on affect (verbal and nonverbal), as well as cognition (thoughts, fantasies, and so forth). The types and components of interpretations will be coded as described by Malan (12).

Variation of Technique Across Treatment Groups

The goal of the video coding system was to identify specific therapist interventions and patient responses in different treatment conditions. Preliminary analyses of certain therapist activities has indicated that this system can demonstrate significant differences among our experimental groups. As shown in Table 3, significant differences between the STDP and BAP group were found on the four variables that have been analyzed.

The number of confrontations varied significantly, with an average of 53.8 per session in the STDP, as compared to an average of 11.2 in the BAP group (p = .007). The number of therapist statements concerning feelings varied from an average of 36.2 per session in the STDP group to only 3.2 per session in the BAP group (p = .002). Similarly, the number of therapist statements concerning nonverbal behavior averaged 6.8 per session in the STDP group and were nonexistent (**x** = 0) in the BAP group (p = .045). The number of statements by the therapist concerning the patient-therapist relationship averaged 16.5 per session in the STDP groups, while the BAP group averaged only 4.0 per session (p = .05).

One often finds that results that are statistically significant may not be clinically relevant. This is not the case here. The differences in techniques make for dramatic contrasts in therapy style, as one can observe by viewing the videotapes of psychotherapy sessions. The evident impact on the patients in each group is very

Table 3. Preliminary Analysis of Differences Between Groups on Therapist Activity Variables*

Variable	Operational Definition	STDP Group	BAP Group	Significance
Confrontation	Frequency of confrontive statements	*X*=53.8 SD 24.4	*X*=11.2 SD 13.7	*p*=.007
Affective Focus	Number of therapist statements concerning feelings	*X*=36.2 *SD*=14.0	*X*=3.2 *SD*=2.4	*p*=.0002
	Number of therapist statements concerning patient's non-verbal behavior	*X*=6.8 *SD*=6.5	*X*=0.0 *SD*=0	*p*=.045
	Number of patient statements concerning feelings	Predicted Values High Coded—not yet analyzed	Low	
	Number of patient behaviors indicating affect (smiling, crying, sighing, fidgeting, lowering eyes, etc.)	Predicted Values High Coded—not yet analyzed	Low	
Cognitive Focus	Number of therapist statements concerning thoughts, fantasies, images, etc.	Predicted Values Low Coded—not yet analyzed	High	
	Number of patient statements concerning thoughts, fantasies, images, etc.	Predicted Values Low Not Yet Coded	High	
Patient-Therapist	Number of statements by therapist concerning relationship	High *X*=16.5 *SD*=11.9	Low *X*=4.0 *SD*=3.3	*p*=.05
Past-Present Links		Predicted Values Low Coded—not yet analyzed	High	

* One tailed tests

different, as well. We anticipate significant differences in patient responses, especially in the category of "experienced affect" across the two groups.

In addition, the two treatment groups presented here look very different from videotapes of long-term psychotherapy. Although the BAP group is less active in several ways than is the STDP group, the BAP group is much more confrontive (for example, 11.2 confrontations per hour) than traditional psychotherapy, which may have no confrontations in a session. Thus, we have preliminary data that support the reliability of the coding schema, as well as the validity of the system for differentiating different forms of brief therapy versus long-term therapy.

SUMMARY

As a result of the clinical and research work of Sifneos, Malan, and Davanloo, the field of psychoanalytically based psychodynamic psychotherapies has acquired a range of techniques that can be readily operationalized and applied to specific homogeneous patient groups with positive and stable outcomes. Our own pilot work—now in the process of being replicated under more rigorous experimental conditions—reinforces some of the clinical hypotheses of Sifneos, Malan, and Davanloo.

It is possible to develop specific techniques that are based on psychoanalytic psychodynamic principles, and that are suited to specific patient problems. In our study, two forms of short-term psychotherapy can be readily taught to therapists of various levels of experience, and their work can be reliably discriminated by blind raters. Both forms of psychotherapy have differential impact on the psychotherapeutic process. The therapy containing a confrontational stance, a focus on affect, and a more intense use of the patient-therapist relationship, leads to a more stormy psychotherapy process. According to clinical lore, this is a necessary precondition for deeper changes in patients suffering from personality disorders.

The analysis of the termination and followup data of our study will allow us to test process-outcome correlations, such as the impact on outcome of the use and nonuse of transference, past-present links, and so forth. These are essential steps in the construction of a theory of psychotherapy.

References

1. Eysenck HJ: The effect of psychotherapy—an evaluation. J Consult Clin Psychol 16:317-324, 1952
2. Smith ML, Glass GV, Miller T: The Benefit of Psychotherapy. Baltimore, The Johns Hopkins University Press, 1980
3. Frank JD, Gliedman LH, Imber SD, et al: Patient expectancies and relearning as factual, determining improvement in psychotherapy. Am J Psychiatry 115:961-968, 1959
4. Strupp HH, Hadley SW: Specific versus non-specific factors in psychotherapy. Arch Gen Psychiatry 36:1125-1126, 1979
5. Weissman MM: The psychological treatment of depression: evidence for the efficacy of psychotherapy alone, in comparison with and in combination with pharmacotherapy. Arch Gen Psychiatry 36:1261-1269, 1979
6. Beck AT: Cognitive therapy of depression: new perspectives, in Depression. Edited by Crayton P. New York, Raven Press, 1983
7. Strupp HH: Success and failure in time-limited psychotherapy. Arch Gen Psychiatry 37:831-841, 1980
8. Beck AT, Ruch AJ, Shaw BF, et al: Cognitive Therapy of Depression. New York, Guilford, 1979
9. Sifneos P: Short-Term Psychotherapy and Emotional Crisis. Cambridge, Harvard University Press, 1972
10. Sifneos P: Short-Term Dynamic Psychotherapy. New York, Plenum Press, 1979

11. Malan DH: A Study of Brief Psychotherapy. New York, Plenum Press, 1963

12. Malan DH: The Frontier of Brief Psychotherapy. New York, Plenum Press, 1976

13. Malan DH: Towards the Validation of Dynamic Psychotherapy. New York, Plenum Press, 1980

14. Davanloo H: Basic Principles and Techniques in Short-Term Dynamic Psychotherapy. New York, Spectrum Publications, 1978

15. Davanloo H: Techniques of short-term dynamic psychotherapy. Psychiatr Clin North Am II (1): April, 1979

16. Davanloo H: Short-Term Dynamic Psychotherapy. New York, Jason Aronson, 1980

17. Weiner IB: Principles of Psychotherapy. New York, John Wiley & Sons, 1976

6

Applicants for Short-Term Dynamic Psychotherapy

Henry Pinsker, M.D.
Peggy Nepps, Psy.D.
Joel Redfield, Ph.D.
Arnold Winston, M.D.

6

Applicants for Short-Term Dynamic Psychotherapy

The indications for psychotherapy and the process of psychotherapy have been extensively described. The outcome of therapies is a topic of great current concern. It seems that remarkably little attention has been directed to the study of the population who seek (but do not necessarily enter) psychotherapy, and to analysis of the way potential patients seek therapists. The National Center for Disease Statistics knew of no recent data on psychiatric outpatients, and no papers describing outpatient populations were found in a computer search of recent literature. One of the few papers on the topic is Lazar's (1) comparison of applicants for treatment at Columbia University Psychoanalytic Clinic in 1971, with those who applied between 1952 and 1959. Lazar concluded that there was an impressive shift away from diagnosis of neurosis and toward diagnosis of personality disorder. Lazar found that the mean age of analytic applicants had decreased (in 1971, 80 percent were under 30) and that women outnumbered men by one and one-half to one. These potential analytic patients were mostly either professionals, white collar workers, or students.

Lazar's sample is obviously select, insofar as it reflects only potential analytic patients. Many people seek and enter a wide variety of outpatient treatments, in private offices as well as in many different types of clinics. Although most mental health facilities routinely collect some data about their applicants and patients for either program evaluation or reports to governing bodies, there are no routinely published statistics. The New York State Office of Mental Health (2) has recently begun one week samplings of patient care in all licensed mental health facilities. The 1981 data is available, but the 1982 and 1983 data has not yet been completely analyzed.

During the 1981 sample week, 36,372 adult visits were reported from all outpatient facilities in New York City. Of these, 63.1 percent were women. Although the State sample includes data on "prescreening interviews," patients in this category in some settings also included applicants for inpatient treatment, so the sample data does not illuminate the question of who applies for outpatient treatment. In this sample, 61.3 percent of the patients were white, 19.4 percent were black, and 17.7 percent were Hispanic.

That the media play an increasingly important role in informing patients about medical matters is widely known. The stereotype among physicians is that people learn about new treatments, or alleged cures, from television or newspapers, and then ask their physicians to provide this treatment or refer them to someone who can. Many individuals do not, however, seek referral, but use what they have learned from the media to make their own arrangements for treatment. Media coverage not only incites some patients to seek "breakthrough" cures for chronic diseases, but it also provides information about selection of psychotherapists and forms of psychotherapy.

The authors had the opportunity to describe the type of patient who responds to media information when Beth Israel Medical Center's Department of Psychiatry was mentioned in an article about short-term dynamic psychotherapy in the New York Times Magazine in November 1982. In conventional journalistic style, ideas and information were expressed by means of quotations from several staff members. The article was conservatively written, and described the tenets of short-term dynamic psychotherapy with emphasis on the importance of the therapist's activity. It did not disparage conventional psychotherapy, nor did it suggest that

Table 1. Identifying Information

Age Range	Percent	Sex	Percent
18–25	10.3	Male	35.4
26–40	55.3	Female	64.6
41–55	24.8		
56–82	9.4		
Marital Status	**Percent**	**Calling Status**	**Percent**
Single	53.6	Early	78.2
Married	24.4	Late	21.8
Previously married	22.2		

this new approach would eclipse other approaches to treatment. Immediately after the article appeared, many people called to inquire about the availability of this treatment. Although the volume of calls slowed after the first month, inquiries that appeared to have been stimulated by the article continued to arrive, although in progressively smaller numbers, over the next two years.

It was decided to study the data collected about these callers to determine whether the potential patients, as a group, were characterized by any identifiable patterns of symptoms or behavior. It should be noted that the New York Times Magazine, which is a section of the Sunday newspaper, is aimed at readers who have at least a college education. In this regard, it does not compete with general interest newspapers or magazines.

It was hypothesized, in terms of demographic data, that the population of applicants would resemble the population of a private practice or of an analytic training clinic; that is, that the applicants would be young and well educated. It was also thought that the presenting problems and the reasons for seeking short-term treatment would correspond to the problems and treatment characteristics mentioned in the article. For example, it was thought that many callers would have been attracted by the possibility of completing treatment with only a moderate investment in time. It was also thought that there might be differences between those who called immediately after reading the article and those who called later.

Table 2. Occupation

Professional/Managerial	31.3 percent
Technical/Blue Collar	20.5 percent
Arts/Media	24.1 percent
Sales/Self-employed	5.9 percent
Not working	18.2 percent

Callers were asked to leave only their name and telephone number, and were told that they would be contacted for telephone screening. These interviews, conducted by several members of the secretarial staff and a few student volunteers, were used to obtain information about age, sex, marital status, occupation, presenting problems, prior treatment, psychiatric history, and reasons for seeking short-term psychotherapy. Answers were either recorded verbatim or were paraphrased. Every caller was told that he or she would be contacted to schedule an evaluation when an opening in the short-term psychotherapy program became available. Those who did not wish to wait, or to accept the uncertainty about whether waiting would result in acceptance into treatment, were offered referrals for conventional psychotherapy.

Data were analyzed from a stratified random sample of those who called between November 22, 1982, and June 30, 1983. The sample was stratified on the basis of calling status; that is, early (before January 31, 1983) or late (after January 31, 1984) with respect to the publication of the article, and according to whether or not they had been accepted for treatment at the time the sample was drawn. The sample consisted of 312 cases out of a total population of 450. The transcripts of the telephone interviews were coded by Dr. Nepps, who is a doctoral-level psychologist, assisted by an undergraduate psychology student. The coding system used was developed in collaboration with Dr. Pinsker, a psychiatrist.

Table 1 displays identifying information about the patient sample. Women made up 64.6 percent of the sample, and 53.6 percent of the callers were single. Only 24.4 percent were currently married. Callers in the age group of 26 to 40 constituted 55.3 percent of the sample. Ten percent were younger than 26; nine

Table 3. Treatment History

Courses of Treatment		Months of Treatment	
0	14.1 percent	<1	23.7 percent
1–2	52.2 percent	1–24	28.8 percent
3–4	29.8 percent	25–60	23.1 percent
5+	3.8 percent	61–240	24.4 percent

Type of Treatment	
Individual psychotherapy	78.5 percent
Couple/Family	7.4 percent
Group	13.8 percent
Other	23.1 percent

percent were older than 55. "Early" callers comprised 78.2 percent of the group.

The occupations of callers are listed in Table 2. Thirty-one percent of the sample held positions classified as professional or managerial. Another 24 percent held jobs in the arts or media, while 20.5 percent claimed technical or blue collar occupations. The unemployed, retired persons, homemakers, and students were all classified as "not working"; they comprised 18.2 percent of the sample.

The previous treatment history of applicants is described in Table 3. Only 14.1 percent had never been in treatment. Another 39 percent said they were in treatment at the time they called. On the basis of subsequent interviews with some of the callers, however, it is suspected that many callers who were in treatment did not disclose this at the time of their telephone interview, making that 39 percent a rather conservative estimate. Fifty-two percent of the callers had only one or two courses of prior treatment, while an additional 34 percent had been in treatment three times or more. Callers were also asked about the duration of previous treatment, and all prior courses were summed for each patient. The mean sum was two years or more for half of the sample; it was less than two years for the other half. Callers were also asked to identify the treatment modalities of their prior care. Individual treatment, possibly in conjunction with other modalities, was reported by 78.5 percent.

Table 4. Presenting Problems

Problem	Percent
Troubled relationships	31.0
Depression	27.6
Self-image	27.6
Anxiety	20.4
Phobias and fears	20.4
Role performance: work	18.0
Withdraws/avoids relationships	17.0
Other	15.0
Lack of direction	13.9
Other behavioral problems	13.9
Physical symptoms	13.3
Can't establish relationships	9.9
Eating	8.5
Anger: excessive	8.2
Affective problem: nonspecific	7.8
Expression of affect	5.8
Passivity	5.8
General relationship problems	5.4
Procrastination	5.4
Compulsions	5.1
Psychosocial stressors: other	4.8
Anger: can't express	4.4
Sexual performance	4.1
Guilt	4.1
Divorce/break-up	4.1
Assertiveness	3.7
Physical illness	2.7
Role performance: school	2.7
Role performance: home	2.4
Grief	2.4
Obsessions	2.0
Other life changes	2.0
Dependency	1.7
Sexual identity	1.7
"Empty nest"	1.4
Other mid-life crisis	1.0
Career change	1.0
Role performance: other	1.0
Perfectionism	0.7
Undefined stress	0.7

Table 5. General Problem Category

Relationship	46.2 percent
Affective	50.3 percent
Behavioral	44.9 percent
Other	73.4 percent

In order to assess psychiatric history, callers were asked about prior psychiatric hospitalization, suicide attempts, and disabling psychiatric symptoms. A positive response to any of these three resulted in the caller being classified as having a history of major impairment. Callers were also asked about the use of psychotropic medications and about drug and alcohol abuse. A quarter of the sample had a history of major impairment or disorder; 27 percent had been prescribed psychotropic medications, and 13 percent admitted past or present substance abuse.

In terms of identifying information, therefore, our prototypical caller was a single woman, between the ages of 26 and 40, who held a professional or managerial job, and who had one or two courses of individual psychotherapy in the past, probably without a major psychiatric disorder or a history of substance abuse. The sample resembles a private practice clientele, or a psychotherapy clinic rather than a hospital clinic.

As noted above, callers were also questioned about their presenting problems. Table 4 shows the frequency data for the 40 categories used to code problems. Because most callers expressed more than one problem, the percentages sum to more than 100. Troubled relationships, depression, and self-image were the most common problem areas, with almost one-third of the callers mentioning each one. These were followed by difficulties with anxiety, phobias, and fears, and with role performance at work. In an effort to facilitate analysis, the problems were condensed into four broad categories. Those who said they had troubled relationships, tended to withdraw from others, or tended to have difficulties seeking others, were described as having "relationship" problems. Those who were depressed, anxious, or troubled by anger, grief, or guilt were categorized as having "affective" problems. Callers who reported phobias, fears, eating problems, compulsions,

Table 6. Reasons for Seeking Short-Term Dynamic Psychotherapy

Previous treatment unsatisfactory	32.1 percent
Attracted to the technique	17.0 percent
Concerns about time	32.7 percent
Need confrontation	28.2 percent
Other	17.9 percent

obsessions, stress, procrastination, lack of assertiveness, and perfectionism were labeled as having "behavioral" difficulties. Finally, the category of "other" problems was used to cover the remaining kinds of difficulties, which included: role performance, psychosocial stressors, self-image, physical symptoms, passivity, dependency, lack of direction, and sexual identity.

Table 5 shows the frequency of problems when classified in this manner. As can be seen, the "other" category accounted for the largest percentage, with 73.4 percent of the callers complaining of these kinds of difficulties. This was followed by affective problems, which were mentioned by 50.3 percent of the callers.

In Table 6, reasons for seeking short-term treatment are listed. Callers were simply asked: "Why do you seek brief treatment?"; many of them volunteered more than one reason. Ten categories of reasons were abstracted for coding purposes, and those ten were condensed into the five categories shown, for purposes of analysis. Of all reasons cited, the category of "previous treatment unsatisfactory," which included such complaints as former care being "too slow"or "lacking vigor," comprised 32.1 percent. An equal percentage stated that they were hopeful that treatment could be completed in a shorter time. The magazine article had emphasized the use of confrontation in short-term dynamic psychotherapy, and 28.2 percent of the callers stated that this was what they felt they needed. The category "attracted to technique" reflects many vague or general responses on the theme of liking what was read in the magazine article and therefore wanting to try it. The remaining 17.9 percent were classified as "other" reasons, and included such motivations as other people's recommendations, liking the idea of being videotaped, and hopes that the treatment would be less expensive than longer therapy.

Table 7. Previous Treatment History and Calling Status

Number of courses	Percent Early	Percent Late
0	67.4	32.6
1–2	86.3	13.8
3–4	69.9	30.1
5+	75.0	25.0

Possible relationships among different variables were analyzed by means of computer assisted chi squares. Table 7 displays the relationship between calling status and treatment history. Those who had already had three or more courses of treatment were more likely to be late callers, as were those who had never been in treatment. Those who described only one or two prior courses were more likely to call early. Another significant difference between early and late callers was that 35.7 percent of the early callers' reasons fell into the category "previous treatment unsatisfactory," while only 19.4 percent of the late callers' did so. Late callers, however, showed a stronger tendency than early callers to cite either "attracted to technique," or "other" as reasons for seeking short-term treatment. This suggests that late callers were less dissatisfied, as well as less specific, in their reasons than were early callers. Early callers were more likely to have affective problems, while late callers were more likely to have relationship problems (but the differences were not statistically significant).

Hypothesized relationships among variables were confirmed at the $p \leq .01$ level in seven cases. Table 8 summarizes these relationships. Three of the seven relationships involved the differences between early callers and late callers that were discussed above. The remaining four relationships suggest the following:

1. Those without major impairment were much more likely than those with major impairment to give as a reason for seeking treatment: problems with relationships, affect, or behavior;

2. Those not currently in treatment were significantly more likely than those in treatment to give these reasons;

3. Those currently in treatment were much more likely than those not in treatment to cite dissatisfaction as a reason;

Table 8. Significant Relationships ($p < .01$)

Date of contact and *Number of previous treatments*
Date of contact and *Previous treatment unsatisfactory*
Date of contact and *Attracted to the technique*
Major impairment and *Other reasons for seeking treatment*
Currently in treatment and *Other reasons*
Currently in treatment and *Previous treatment unsatisfactory*
Attracted to the technique and *Other problems*

Table 9. Occupation and Reasons for Seeking Treatment

Occupation	Percent concerned about time	Percent needing confrontation
Professional/Managerial	31.3	25.0
Technical/Blue Collar	34.9	27.0
Arts/Media	28.4	37.8
Sales/Self-employed	27.8	27.8
Not working	36.5	17.3

4. Those with problems classified as "other" were more likely than those with more specific complaints to give "attracted to technique" as a reason.

It appears that those in arts and media were disproportionately interested in confrontation in comparison to the other occupational groups, according to the analysis of reasons for treatment by occupation (Table 9). This table also shows a nonsignificant trend toward greater concerns about time among those who were not working than among other groups.

Chi squares performed with many other variable pairs failed to yield differences. Early and late callers did not vary when it came to age, occupation, behavioral or affective problems, need for confrontation, or concerns about time. Occupation was not related to the number of previous courses of treatment, dissatisfaction with previous treatment, attraction to short-term technique, other reasons, or type of problems. Current treatment status was unrelated to time concerns or need for confrontation. Surprisingly, neither major impairment nor substance abuse status predicted number of prior treatments, previous dissatisfaction, attraction to short-term, time concerns, need for confrontation, or relationship or affective problems.

The patients attracted to short-term dynamic therapy by the magazine article were young, but not as young as were the 1971 applicants for treatment at a psychoanalytic clinic. Most of the callers indicated that they had more than one problem, and the problems reported were diverse. The most frequently mentioned problems were troubled relationships, depression, and negative self image. The typical patient was an unmarried woman whose age was between 26 and 40, employed, but dissatisfied with some aspect of work performance; able to form relationships, but not satisfied with them; troubled by symptoms of depression and anxiety. Classical neuroses, as in the 1971 analytic candidate study, were not numerous. The report of phobias or fears by 20.4 percent may be related to the fact that the magazine article had indicated that phobia was one of the conditions for which this treatment was well suited.

Eighty-five percent of the callers had experience with psychotherapy, and one-fourth of them reported more than five years of treatment. Just as the callers' problems were diverse, so were the reasons for calling (that is, reason for wanting this treatment). The majority of reasons fell into the category of "other," or the nonspecific "attracted to the technique." It was notable that economy of time and money was not a prominent reason. The potential patients were broadly dissatisfied with their lives, and were also dissatisfied with their previous treatment. For the most part, they were seeking effective therapy, not economy or efficiency.

The ideal psychotherapy patient, if dissatisfied with the therapy, brings this up for examination. It seems probable that many who called to request this new treatment were inclined to change therapists. Our data do not provide a precise picture of this because the callers were not pressed to reveal whether the previous treatment they described was current. Increasingly, patients of all sorts perceive themselves as consumers. Whether we like it or not, many patients see their psychotherapists in pragmatic terms, and are willing to replace them with what they hope will be more effective "models."

Although the magazine article emphasized confrontation of defenses, it is possible that some of the callers who specified that they needed confrontation mistakenly equated confrontation with interaction or directiveness, since many had complained that their previous treatment lacked vigor. Of course, we cannot determine from this data the extent of potential patients' understanding of the article.

Despite the sense that previous treatment was not effective, however, these callers appear to have remained hopeful that psychotherapy has the potential to help them, and they are ready to try again. Almost every therapist has patients who have been in treatment before; few therapists know when their former patients enter treatment with someone else. Some patients seek a new therapist because previous treatment has not been sufficiently effective; others seek a new therapist because previous success in treatment has convinced them that the method is useful.

Our study of information obtained in initial telephone interviews of inquirers about short-term dynamic psychotherapy failed to point up major differences between men and women, old and young, those who had long treatment history and those who did not. Those who called within the first ten weeks after the article appeared were more likely to express specific dissatisfaction with previous treatment, which in many instances was on-going, while those who called later were less specific in their reasons.

To what extent does this sample of responders to the article resemble the population of psychotherapy patients? With the possible exception of the 24 percent who worked in arts or media, which may be idiosyncratic to New York, we believe that the pool of patients is similar to a typical psychotherapy practice. The sample showed some resemblance to Lazar's description of analytic candidates in terms of occupation and diffuse symptoms. The ratio of men to women resembled aggregated data from all New York City facilities.

The fact that one-fourth of the callers may have been seriously impaired, or at least impaired enough to be unsuitable for the treatment described in the article, is not surprising. A large number of suffering people read a message of hope for finding solutions to their own problems into any news item or any public statement about a new therapeutic technique.

Medical progress is a significant part of the news offered to the public by way of magazines, newspapers, and television. Little notice has been given to the practice of intentional use of news media by physicians as a means of soliciting patients. Advertising is now ethically permissible, provided it is modest and inoffensive. Those who need a continuing supply of patients, as those who conduct drug trials, must often recruit continuously, often employing advertisements. Increasingly, the techniques of public relations are employed. Press releases are sent to newspapers and efforts are made to "plant" news items or to arrange television interviews.

The effort to provide appropriate treatment for those who need it requires that attention be directed to systems of communication, to the public as well as to physicians, about treatment techniques and indications for these techniques, expressed in realistic language. Responsibility to patients requires psychotherapists to pay attention to those whose hopes are raised by publicity to the point that they initiate a request for help.

References

1. Lazar ND: Nature and significance of changes in patients in a psychoanalytic clinic. Psychoanal Q 42:579–600, 1973

2. New York State Office of Mental Health. Survey of Patient Characteristics 1981, Vol. I. Albany, New York, New York State Office of Mental Health, 1983